The Guru Method

General Chemistry

For information contact:

GSMS Education Pty Ltd
P.O Box 3848
Marsfield NSW
2122
Australia

General Chemistry - The Guru Method

Chemistry represents 40% of the questions that are asked in the GAMSAT. Like all other questions in section III, the information required to answer the questions are generally contained in the passage. However, possessing a background in chemistry will give you an advantage. Like physics, chemistry is a "thinking" science but with some key differences.

My high school science teacher once asked me "What do you prefer, a subject that asks you to remember the application of details or the application of concepts?"

"What's the difference?" I replied.

That's the difference between physics and chemistry.

Chemistry is more about (although not strictly true) the application of details. This manual will provide you with some knowledge of chemistry, as well as the skills you need to answer GAMSAT chemistry questions. Most topics are divided into three parts. The "Quick Facts" will give you basic knowledge of the topic. "Practice Questions" will test you on your knowledge of the subject material. "GAMSAT Style Questions" contain questions that have been written in the style and difficulty level of the GAMSAT. In some topics I have skipped parts because I feel that they do not contribute to your ability to perform in the GAMSAT. This manual is not a substitute for chemistry textbook. If you have trouble grasping the concepts mentioned in this book, you should consult a chemistry textbook. Use this manual as a guide to studying for the GAMSAT, not studying chemistry.

Table of Contents

Chapter 1: Periodic Table

Key Concepts: Periodic Table

The periodic table is an arrangement of the elements based on increasing atomic number that shows relationships between element properties. A large amount of information can be obtained from the periodic table. The table below has been coded to differentiate various groups of elements within the table that have similar properties.

Periodic Table of Elements

Group 1	Group 2	Group 3	Group 4	Group 5	Group 6	Group 7	Group 8	Group 9	Group 10	Group 11	Group 12	Group 13	Group 14	Group 15	Group 16	Group 17	Group 18
1 H 1.0																	2 He 4.0
3 Li 6.9	4 Be 9.0											5 B 10.8	6 C 12.0	7 N 14.0	8 O 16.0	9 F 19.0	10 Ne 20.2
11 Na 23.0	12 Mg 24.3											13 Al 27.0	14 Si 28.1	15 P 31.0	16 S 32.1	17 Cl 35.5	18 Ar 40.0
19 K 39.1	20 Ca 40.1	21 Sc 45.0	22 Ti 47.9	23 V 50.9	24 Cr 52.0	25 Mn 54.9	26 Fe 55.8	27 Co 58.9	28 Ni 58.7	29 Cu 63.5	30 Zn 65.4	31 Ga 69.7	32 Ge 72.6	33 As 74.9	34 Se 79.0	35 Br 79.9	36 Kr 83.8
37 Rb 85.5	38 Sr 87.6	39 Y 88.9	40 Zr 91.2	41 Nb 92.9	42 Mo 95.9	43 Tc 98.9	44 Ru 101.1	45 Rh 102.9	46 Pd 106.4	47 Ag 107.9	48 Cd 112.4	49 In 114.8	50 Sn 118.7	51 Sb 121.8	52 Te 127.6	53 I 126.9	54 Xe 131.3
55 Cs 132.9	56 Ba 137.3	71 Lu 175.0	72 Hf 178.5	73 Ta 180.9	74 W 183.8	75 Re 186.2	76 Os 190.2	77 Ir 192.2	78 Pt 195.1	79 Au 197.0	80 Hg 200.6	81 Tl 204.4	82 Pb 207.7	83 Bi 209.0	84 Po 209.0	85 At 210.0	86 Rn 222.0
87 Fr 223.0	88 Ra 226.0	103 Lr 260.1	104 Rf 261.1	105 Db 262.1	106 Sg 263.1	107 Bh 262.0	108 Hs 265.0	109 Mt 266.0	110 Ds 269.0	111 Rg 272.0	112 Uub 277.0	113 Uut 284.0	114 Unq 289.0	115 Uup 288.0	116 Uuh 292		

57 La 138.9	58 Ce 140.1	59 Pr 140.9	60 Nd 144.2	61 Pm 144.9	62 Sm 150.4	63 Eu 152.0	64 Gd 157.2	65 Tb 158.9	66 Dy 162.5	67 Ho 164.9	68 Er 167.3	69 Tm 168.9	70 Yb 170.3
89 Ac 227.0	90 Th 232.0	91 Pa 231.0	92 U 238.0	93 Np 237.0	94 Pu 244.1	95 Am 243.1	96 Cm 247.1	97 Bk 247.1	98 Cf 251.1	99 Es 252.1	100 Fm 257.1	101 Md 258.1	102 No 259.1

Metals
- Alkali Metals
- Alkaline-Earth Metals
- Transition Metals
- Other Metals

Nonmetals
- Halogens
- Noble Gases
- Other Nonmetals

Other
- Hydrogen
- Semiconductors (Metalloids)

In addition to providing information regarding certain physical properties of the different elements, each box within the table contains the elemental symbol and two numbers. These numbers correspond to the atomic number and atomic mass of the element.

Tip: **Know this figure. This is fundamental.**

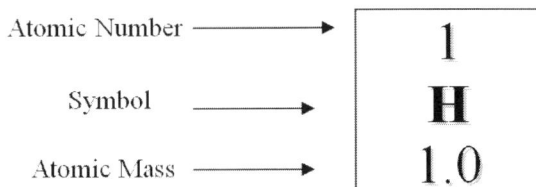

Atomic Number ⟶

Symbol ⟶

Atomic Mass ⟶

| 1 |
| **H** |
| 1.0 |

Key Concepts: General Trends within the Periodic Table

The periodic table is set up in such a way that certain trends with respect to properties can be predicted when moving across the table from left to right, or within a particular group when moving from top to bottom. These periodic properties are directly related to the electron configuration of the atoms. Recall that the capacity of the first electron orbital (the s orbital) is two electrons and for the second orbital (the p orbital) the capacity is six. Elements need a full outer electron orbital in order to be stable and therefore, will form bonds with themselves or other elements to achieve this state.

Atomic Number

The atomic number is equal to the number of protons in an atom, and the number of electrons in a neutral atom. This number defines what element it is and determines the chemical behaviour of that element. For example carbon atoms have six protons, hydrogen atoms have one, and oxygen atoms have eight.

Atomic Mass

The atomic mass is the average mass of an element in atomic mass units (amu). Individual atoms always have an integer number of atomic mass units, however; the atomic mass on the periodic table is stated as a decimal number because it is an average of the different isotopes of that element. The average number of neutrons for an element can be found by subtracting the number of protons (atomic number) from the atomic mass. The atomic mass increases with increasing atomic number.

Atomic Radius

The atomic radius of an element is half of the distance between the centres of two atoms of that element that are just touching each other. Generally, the atomic radius decreases across a period from left to right and increases down a given group.

Ionization Energy

The ionization energy is the minimum amount of energy necessary to remove an electron from an atom or ion in the gas phase. Normally, it will be the valence electrons that are removed first since they are furthest away from the nucleus and thus have less attraction to it. Once the valence electrons have all been removed, a large increase in ionization energy will be necessary to remove another electron. Ionization energy is influenced by atomic radius, in that smaller atoms will have higher ionization energies since they tend to hold on more tightly to their electrons. In addition, electrons in the *p* orbital are easier to remove than those in the *s* orbital, and unpaired electrons are easier to remove than paired.

Electron Affinity

Electron affinity reflects the ability of an atom to accept an electron. Atoms with stronger effective nuclear charge will have a greater electron affinity. With respect to the electron affinities of certain groups in the periodic table, certain generalizations can be made. The Group 2 elements, the alkaline earths, have low electron affinity values. These elements are relatively stable because they have filled *s* orbitals. Group 17 elements, the halogens, have high electron affinities because only need one additional electron to completely fill their outer shell. Group 1B elements, noble gases, have electron affinities near zero, since each atom possesses a stable octet and will not accept an electron readily. Elements of other groups have low electron affinities.

Electronegativity

Electronegativity is a measure of the attraction of an atom for the electrons in a chemical bond. An atom with a high electronegativity will have a greater attraction for bonding electrons. Electronegativity and ionization energy are related in that electrons with low ionization energies have low electronegativities because their nuclei do not exert a strong attractive force on electrons. Elements with high ionization energies have high electronegativities due to the strong pull exerted on electrons by the nucleus. Within a group, the electronegativity will decrease with an increase in atomic number. This is due to the increase in distance between the valence electron and nucleus (greater atomic radius). An example of an element with low electronegativity is caesium; one with high electronegative is fluorine.

Electron Configuration

One more very important property of the periodic table is its ability to give you the electron configuration within an atom. There are four possible orbitals that electrons will be within a molecule; these are designated by *s*, *p*, *d*, and *f*. 2, 6, 10, and 14 are the number of electrons that are needed to fill each respectively. The first orbital level only has a *s*; the second has a *s* and *p*; the third has *s*, *p*, and *d*; all subsequent level have *s*, *p*, *d*. and *f*.

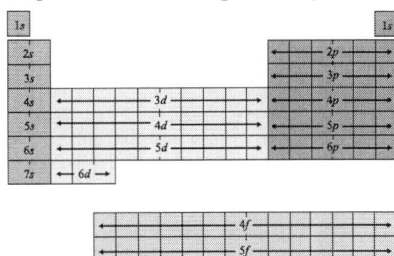

The above table shows which orbital will be the outer orbital for each atom and the order which the orbitals are filled. Each row in the table corresponds to different level.

—> *Quick Facts: Periodic Table Trends*

1 Moving left to right in the table
   o Decrease in atomic radius
   o Increase in ionization energy
   o Increase in electronegativity
   o Increase in atomic number
   o Increase in atomic mass

2 Moving Top to Bottom
   o Increase in atomic radius
   o Decrease in ionization energy
   o Decrease in electronegativity
   o Increase in atomic number
   o Increase in atomic mass

Key Concepts: Chemical Properties

Metals – form cations when in solutions

- Shiny 'metallic' appearance
- Solids at room temperature (except mercury)
- High melting points
- High densities
- Large atomic radii
- Low ionization energies
- Low electronegativities
- Usually, high deformation
- Malleable
- Ductile
- Thermal conductors
- Electrical conductors

Types of metals

Alkali Metals

- Lower densities than other metals
- One loosely bound valence electron
- Largest atomic radii in their periods
- Low ionization energies
- Low electronegativities
- Highly reactive

Alkaline-earth metals

- Two electrons in the outer shell
- Low electron affinities
- Low electronegativities
- Readily form divalent cations

Transition Metals

- Low ionization energies
- Positive oxidation states
- Very hard
- High melting points
- High boiling points
- High electrical conductivity
- Malleable
- Five d orbitals become more filled, from left to right on periodic table

Non-metals –

These elements do not exhibit the characteristics of metals. These elements, in general, are poor conductors and have a high electronegativity.

- High ionization energies
- High electronegativities
- Poor thermal conductors
- Poor electrical conductors
- Brittle solids
- Little or no metallic lustre
- Gain electrons easily

Types of non-metals

Halogens

- Very high electronegativities
- Seven valence electrons (one short of a stable octet)
- Highly reactive, especially with alkali metals and alkaline earths

Noble Gases

- Relatively non-reactive
- Complete valence shell
- High ionization energies
- Very low electronegativities
- Low boiling points (all gases at room temperature)

Others
Semiconductors (metalloids)

- Electronegativities between those of metals and non-metals
- Ionization energies between those of metals and non-metals
- Possess some characteristics of metals/some of non-metals
- Reactivity depends on properties of other elements in reaction
- Often make good semiconductors

Hydrogen

- Smallest of any element
- Exists as a gas at room temperature
- Contains a positive charge and only one electron
- Forms ionic compounds with metals
- Forms molecular compounds with non-metals

Illustrative Question: The Periodic Table

Use the periodic table given to answer the following questions.

Atomic number

1. How many protons are in the following element?

    Hg

Atomic mass

2. Which element of the pair has the greater atomic mass?

    Mn or Ir

Ionization Energy

3. Which element of the pair will have the higher ionization energy?

    Cs or Ba

Electronegativity

4. List the following elements in order of increasing electronegativity.

    Mg, Sr, Ra, Be

Electron configuration

5. Write the electron configurations for the following elements (use diagram in the electron configuration section to assist you).

    As

Solutions

1. Find Hg on the periodic table, recall that the atomic number is the number of protons in an atom. If you look in group 12, you will find Hg with an atomic number of 80, so the answer is 80.

2. Recall that as the atomic number increases so does the atomic mass of an element. In addition, atomic number increases in a row from left to right and in a column from top to bottom. In this case, Mn has a lower atomic number than Ir (25 vs. 77). So, Ir will have the greater atomic mass.

3. Recall that ionization energy increases from left to right and decreases from top to bottom. In this case Cs is further left than Ba. So Ba will have the higher ionization energy. This is because Ba has a pair of electrons in its outer electron shell so it is more difficult to remove an electron from a pair than only a single electron.

4. Recall that electronegativity increases from left to right and decreases from top to bottom so the order of increasing electronegativity would be Ra < Sr < Mg < Be.

5. Using the diagram, just follow the periodic table starting with the top left, go across the row and fill the orbitals until you reach the end of a row, then start on the next row back on the left hand side, the number of electrons that fill the orbitals should equal the atomic number of the element. The atomic number of As is 33, so starting at the left, the first row is $1s$, the next row is $2s$, then $2p$, the next row is $3s$, then $3p$, the next row is $4s$, then $3d$, then $4p$ – this is where you will find As. So remembering that s orbital can have 2 electrons, the p can have 6, the d can have 10, and the f can have 14, fill the orbitals in order. (Note, the last orbital will not be completely filled).

$1s^2 2s^2 2p^6 3s^2 3p^6 4s^2 3d^{10} 4p^3$

To check, add up the electrons 2+2+6+2+6+2+10+3 = 33 – which is the atomic number of As.

Getting to Know the Topic:

Now, try a few on your own.

Atomic number
How many protons are in each of the following elements?
(i) Kr (ii) Fe (iii) Os

Atomic mass
Which element of the pair has the greater atomic mass?
(i) Cr or Ni (ii) V or W (iii) Si or Ge (iv) K or F (v) Se or Sn

Ionization Energy
Which element of the pair will have the higher ionization energy?
(i) Na or Mg (ii) Ca or Sr (iii) Cl or Ar (iv) Kr or Ne

Electronegativity
List the following elements in order of increasing electronegativity.
- (i)   Cl, F, I, Br, At
- (ii) Ge, As, Se, Ga
- (iii) Si, Sn, Cl, P, S

Electron configuration
Write the electron configurations for the following elements (use diagram in electron configuration section to assist you).
- (i)   La
- (ii) Se
- (iii) Ar
- (iv) Pu

Solutions

Atomic number
  (i)   36
  (ii) 26
  (iii) 76

Atomic mass
  (i)   Ni
  (ii) W
  (iii) Ge
  (iv) K
  (v)   Sn

Ionization energy
  (i)   Mg
  (ii) Ca
  (iii) Ar
  (iv) Ne

Electronegativity
  (i)   At, I, Br, Cl, F
  (ii) Ga, Ge, As, Se
  (iii) Sn, Si, P, S, Cl

Electron Configuration
  (i)   La (57) - $1s^2 2s^2 2p^6 3s^2 3p^6 4s^2 3d^{10} 4p^6 5s^2 4d^{10} 5p^6 6s^2 4f^1$
  (ii) Se (34) - $1s^2 2s^2 2p^6 3s^2 3p^6 4s^2 3d^{10} 4p^4$
  (iii) Ar (18) - $1s^2 2s^2 2p^6 3s^2 3p^6$
  (iv) Pu (94) - $1s^2 2s^2 2p^6 3s^2 3p^6 4s^2 3d^{10} 4p^6 5s^2 4d^{10} 5p^6 6s^2 4f^{14} 5d^{10} 6p^6 7s^2 5f^6$

GAMSAT Style Questions

Question 1-4

The electrons of an element can occupy 4 different electron orbitals: s, p, d, and f. 2, 6, 10, and 14 electrons can enter each orbital respectively. The number of electrons in the outer orbital, known as valence electrons, dictates how that element will form bonds. Electrons fill up the orbitals in a specific order, s, then p, then d, then f. Each shell consists of a combination of the orbitals. When n=1 the shell only contains an s orbital, n= 2 contains the s and the p, n = 3 contains s, p, and d, and n = 4 and above has s, p, d, and f.

Periodic Table of Elements

1																	2
H 1.0																	He 4.0
3 Li 6.9	4 Be 9.0											5 B 10.8	6 C 12.0	7 N 14.0	8 O 16.0	9 F 19.0	10 Ne 20.2
11 Na 23.0	12 Mg 24.3											13 Al 27.0	14 Si 28.1	15 P 31.0	16 S 32.1	17 Cl 35.5	18 Ar 40.0
19 K 39.1	20 Ca 40.1	21 Sc 45.0	22 Ti 47.9	23 V 50.9	24 Cr 52.0	25 Mn 54.9	26 Fe 55.8	27 Co 58.9	28 Ni 58.7	29 Cu 63.5	30 Zn 65.4	31 Ga 69.7	32 Ge 72.6	33 As 74.9	34 Se 79.0	35 Br 79.9	36 Kr 83.8
37 Rb 85.5	38 Sr 87.6	39 Y 88.9	40 Zr 91.2	41 Nb 92.9	42 Mo 95.9	43 Te 98.9	44 Ru 101.1	45 Rh 102.9	46 Pd 106.4	47 Ag 107.9	48 Cd 112.4	49 In 114.8	50 Sn 118.7	51 Sb 121.8	52 Te 127.6	53 I 126.9	54 Xe 131.3
55 Cs 132.9	56 Ba 137.3	71 Lu 175.0	72 Hf 178.5	73 Ta 180.9	74 W 183.8	75 Re 186.2	76 Os 190.2	77 Ir 192.2	78 Pt 195.1	79 Au 197.0	80 Hg 200.6	81 Tl 204.4	82 Pb 207.7	83 Bi 209.0	84 Po 209.0	85 At 210.0	86 Rn 222.0
87 Fr 223.0	88 Ra 226.0	103 Lr 260.1	104 Rf 261.1	105 Db 262.1	106 Sg 263.1	107 Bh 262.1	108 Hs 265.0	109 Mt 266.0	110 Ds 269.0	111 Rg 272.0	112 Uub 277	113 Uut 284.0	114 Uuq 289.0	115 Uup 288.0			

57 La 138.9	58 Ce 140.1	59 Pr 140.9	60 Nd 144.2	61 Pm 144.9	62 Sm 150.4	63 Eu 152.0	64 Gd 157.2	65 Tb 158.9	66 Dy 162.5	67 Ho 164.9	68 Er 167.3	69 Tm 168.9	70 Yb 170.3
89 Ac 227.0	90 Th 232.0	91 Pa 231.0	92 U 238.0	93 Np 237.0	94 Pu 244.1	95 Am 243.1	96 Cm 247.1	97 Bk 247.1	98 Cf 251.1	99 Es 252.1	100 Fm 257.1	101 Md 258.1	102 No 259.1

1. Given the section of the periodic table above, what would be the electron configuration for chlorine?

    A. $1s^2 1p^6 1d^9$

    B. $1s^2 2s^2 2p^6 3s^7$

    C. $1s^2 2p^6 2s^2 3s^2 3p^5$

    D. $1s^2 2s^2 2p^6 3s^2 3p^5$

2. The transition metals that fall in between the sections of the periodic table above have a *d* orbital as their valence orbital. This orbital is in the n-1 shell. Ag has an atomic number of 47. What would be the configuration of its outer orbital?

    A. $4d^9$

    B. $5d^9$

    C. $4d^7$

    D. $5d^7$

3. Chlorine will form a bond with which element in a 1:1 ratio?

    A. Silicone

    B. Magnesium

    C. Caesium

    D. Neon

4. Which element has the largest atomic radius?

    A. Hydrogen

    B. Fluorine

    C. Francium

    D. Radon

Solution

Question 1

STEP 1 = > What do you need to determine to solve the problem?
You need to determine the electron configuration for chlorine.

STEP 2 = > What relevant data provided in this problem is necessary in order to answer the question?
You are provided with a section of the periodic table that shows shells and valence orbitals. In addition, you are told that 2 electrons will fill an *s* orbital, 6 will fill a *p*, 10 will fill a *d*, and 14 will fill an *f*. You are also told that the n=1 shell has only the *s* orbital, n=2 has *s* and *p*, n= 3 has *s*, *p* and *d*, and n=4 and above has *s*, *p*, *d*, *f*. When you find chlorine on the periodic table (Cl), you see that its atomic number is 17, so there are 17 electrons.

STEP 3 = > Use the relevant data to solve the question
When you find chlorine on the periodic table (Cl), you see that its atomic number is 17, so there are 17 electrons. When you look to the left of the row containing Cl, you see that the outer shell will be n=3, and when you look at the top of the column, you see that the shell will be a p^5. So, fill in the orbitals following the rules and you get answer D.

Question 2

STEP 1 = > What do you need to determine to solve the problem?
You need to determine the electron configuration of the outer orbital of Ag.

STEP 2 = > What relevant data provided in this problem is necessary in order to answer the question?
You are given the atomic number of Ag (47); you are told that the transition metals have d outer orbitals and which fill in the n-1 shell. In addition, you have all the information mentioned in the solution to question 1.

STEP 3 = > Use the relevant data to solve the question
You know that you have 47 electrons, so looking at the section of the table, you see that atomic number 47 will fall in the n= 5 row, 2 spaces back from In. You know that the d orbital can contain 10 electrons, so the last column of the transition metals will be d^{10} and the next to last will be d^9 (the row containing Ag). The shell will be n-1 = 5-1 = 4. So, the outer orbital of Ag is $4d^9$. Answer A.

Question 3

STEP 1 = > What do you need to determine to solve the problem?
You need to determine which element will bond in a 1:1 ratio with Cl.

STEP 2 = > What relevant data provided in this problem is necessary in order to answer the question?
You are given a partial periodic table. It shows that Cl has an s^2p^5 outer shell.

STEP 3 = > Use the relevant data to solve the question
Atoms want a full outer shell consisting of 8 electrons, Cl has 7, so it needs one more. Silicone (Si) has 4 electrons to donate, so it would need to bond to 4 Cl atoms. Magnesium (Mg) has 2 electrons, it would need 2 Cl. Caesium (Cs) has only 1 electron so it would form CsCl in a 1:1 ratio, the answer is C. Neon is a noble gas so it is unreactive and will not bond with Cl.

Question 4

STEP 1 = > What do you need to determine to solve the problem?
You need to determine which element has the largest atomic radius.

STEP 2 = > What relevant data provided in this problem is necessary in order to answer the question?
You are given a section of the periodic table and information about how electrons fill the orbitals. As you go from top to bottom on the table, the number of orbital shells increases.

STEP 3 = > Use the relevant data to solve the question
If you recall from the quick facts, moving from left to right on the periodic table results in a decrease in atomic radius, and moving from top to bottom results in an increase in atomic radius. Therefore the answer is C Francium (Fr).

Chapter 2: **Oxidation State**

Key Concepts: Oxidation Numbers and Redox Reactions

Fundamentally, redox reactions are concerned with the transfer of electrons between species. They are a matched set, in other words, you will not have an oxidation reaction without a reduction reaction occurring at the same time. Each reaction by itself is called a half reaction since you need two half reactions to form a complete redox reaction. When writing redox reactions, typically the electrons are explicitly noted. For example:

$$Cu\ (s) \rightarrow Cu^{2+}\ (aq) + 2e^-$$

What this reaction is saying is that solid copper (which has no charge) is being oxidized (losing electrons) to form a copper ion with a +2 charge. It is important to note that there must be a balance between both sides of the equation, thus since the copper ion has a positive charge of 2, 2 electrons must also be present on the right side of the equation in order to result in an overall neutral charge like that on the left side of the equation. The e^- indicates a free electron, so $2e^-$ means that there are two free electrons available for some other function, namely the reduction of some other species in another half reaction. For instance, here a silver ion is reduced by these two electrons to solid silver.

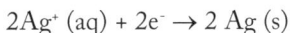

$$2Ag^+\ (aq) + 2e^- \rightarrow 2\ Ag\ (s)$$

When the two half reactions are combined, you get a redox reaction. Note that the free electrons on each side of the equation cancel each other out.

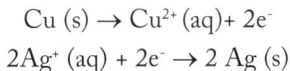

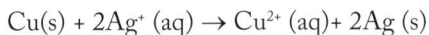

$$Cu\ (s) \rightarrow Cu^{2+}\ (aq) + 2e^-$$
$$2Ag^+\ (aq) + 2e^- \rightarrow 2\ Ag\ (s)$$

$$Cu(s) + 2Ag^+\ (aq) \rightarrow Cu^{2+}\ (aq) + 2Ag\ (s)$$

If a chemical causes another substance to be oxidized, it is called an **oxidizing agent**. Here, Ag^+ is the oxidizing agent since it causes $Cu(s)$ to lose electrons. A chemical that causes another substance to be reduced is called a **reducing agent**. In this case, $Cu(s)$ is the reducing agent since it causes Ag^+ to gain electrons.

The oxidation number of an element indicates the number of electrons lost, gained, or shared as a result of chemical bonding. The change in the oxidation state of a species lets you know if it has undergone oxidation or reduction.

Oxidation can be defined as "an increase in oxidation number". In other words, if a species starts out at one oxidation state and ends up in a higher oxidation state it has undergone oxidation. The species has lost electrons.
Conversely,

Reduction can be defined as "a decrease in oxidation number". Any species whose oxidation number is lowered during the course of a reaction has undergone a reduction. The species has gained electrons.

During a reaction, the substance that brings about the oxidation of another species is known as the oxidizing agent. This species has been reduced. The substance that brings about the reduction of another species is known as the reducing agent. This species has been oxidized.

Balancing Redox reactions
A redox reaction is one in which one species is oxidized while the other is reduced. In order to idenitfy oxidation states within this type of reaction, it is best to split the reaction into two half reactions, the oxidation reaction and the reduction reaction. Then, balance the two halves and finally, add them together again. Take the following example.

Copper metal is added to concentrated nitric acid

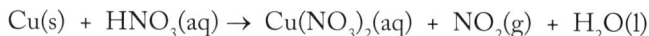

$$Cu(s) + HNO_3(aq) \rightarrow Cu(NO_3)_2(aq) + NO_2(g) + H_2O(l)$$

First divide the equation into half-reactions (notice that the copper is going from a 0 oxidation state to 2+ which is oxidation, and some of the nitrogen is being reduced from 5+ in the nitrate ion to 4+ in the nitrogen dioxide).

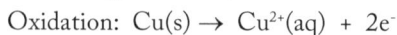

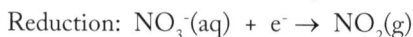

Oxidation: $Cu(s) \rightarrow Cu^{2+}(aq) + 2e^-$
Reduction: $NO_3^-(aq) + e^- \rightarrow NO_2(g)$

Next, balance each half-reaction with respect to atoms first, then with respect to electrons.

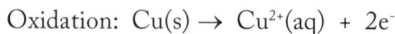

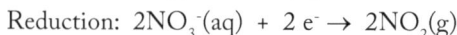

Oxidation: $Cu(s) \rightarrow Cu^{2+}(aq) + 2e^-$
Reduction: $2NO_3^-(aq) + 2e^- \rightarrow 2NO_2(g)$

Notice that there are oxygen atoms in the reduction step that are not balanced. When this occurs, add water molecules on the right in order to balance the total oxygens on the left. Next, to balance the hydrogen atoms, add hydrogen ions on the left.

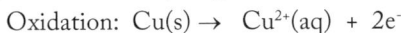

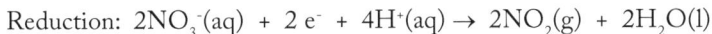

$$\text{Oxidation: } Cu(s) \rightarrow Cu^{2+}(aq) + 2e^-$$
$$\text{Reduction: } 2NO_3^-(aq) + 2e^- + 4H^+(aq) \rightarrow 2NO_2(g) + 2H_2O(l)$$

Finally, add the two half-reactions together cancelling the electrons which are now equal on each side of the arrow.

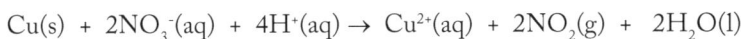

$$Cu(s) + 2NO_3^-(aq) + 4H^+(aq) \rightarrow Cu^{2+}(aq) + 2NO_2(g) + 2H_2O(l)$$

This is what is called the **Net Ionic Equation**. There should always be the same number of electrons lost by the substance that is oxidized which is gained by the substance that is reduced, so that when the two halves are added, the electrons should cancel each other out.

Note: Redox reactions are extremely important in electrochemical cells, and you will need to understand this topic in order to work the problems that will be presented later in the electrochemistry section.

Key Concepts: Rules for assigning Oxidation states

For a monatomic ion, the O.S is the charge on the ion. For a covalently bonded atom, the O.S is the charge on an atom calculated by assigning both electrons of a shared pair to the more electronegative atom. Rules to assign the oxidation states to atoms in ions or molecules:

1. Each pure element has an oxidation state of zero.

    Thus, $Fe(s)$, $N_2(g)$, $P_4(s)$ and $S_8(s)$, are all in the zero oxidation state.

2. In monatomic ions, the O.S. of the element is equal to the charge on the ion. Thus, the O.S. of iron is +3 in the Fe^{3+} ion, and +2 for the Fe^{2+}ion. For Cl^- it is -1 and the O.S. of sulfide S^{2-} is -2.

3. The O.S. of hydrogen in any compound in which it is combined with another element is +1, except in the metallic hydrides such as LiH or CaH_2 where the CaH_2 where the O.S. of H is − 1.

4. The O.S. of oxygen in any compound in which it is combined with another element is – 2, except in the peroxide (BaO_2, Na_2O_2, H_2O_2) where it is -1 and in superoxides (KO_2, CsO_2) where it is – 1/2 and in oxygen difluoride (OF_2) where it is +2.

5. The O.S. of alkali metals in compounds is + 1 and that of alkaline earth metals it is +2.

6. In covalent compounds not involving hydrogen or oxygen, the more electronegative element is assigned its common negative oxidation state. Thus chlorine is assigned – 1 O.S. and sulfur the – 2 O.S.

7. The algebraic sum of the oxidation number of all the atoms combined in a molecule or complex ion must equal the net charge on the molecule or ion.

Oxidation number can be zero, positive or negative, integer or a fraction. A raise in the oxidation state is an oxidation and a lowering of the oxidation state is a reduction.

→ Quick Facts: Balancing redox reactions

- Divide the equation into two half reactions: an oxidation and a reduction half reaction
- Balance these two half reactions
  - o Balance all elements except H and O
  - o Balance O by adding water
  - o Balance H by adding H^+
  - o Balance charges by adding e^-
- Multiply each half reaction by an integer so that the number of e^- lost in one half equals the number gained in the other half
- Combine the half reactions and cancel out identical species from each side
- Ad OH^- to each side until all H^+ is gone and then cancel again

→ *Quick Facts:* **Assigning Oxidation Number**

1. For atoms in their elemental form, the oxidation number is 0
2. For ions, the oxidation number is equal to their charge
3. For hydrogen, the number is usually +1, but in some cases it is -1
4. For oxygen, the number is usually -2
5. The sum of the oxidation number of all atoms in the molecule or ion is equal to its total charge

Illustrative Question: Oxidation Number

Calculate the oxidation state of the underlined atom in the following molecules/ions.
$\underline{Mn}O_4^-$

Solution

Recall that in calculating the oxidation state, The O.S. of oxygen in any compound in which it is combined with another element is -2, except in the peroxide (BaO_2, Na_2O_2, H_2O_2) where it is -1 and in superoxides (KO_2, CsO_2) where it is $-1/2$ and in oxygen difluoride (OF_2) where it is +2. So, since you know that the oxidation state of O in this case is -2, and you know the overall charge on the molecule is -1, you can write an algebraic expression to figure out the O.S. of Mn.

Let x = the oxidation state of Mn.
Then;
$x + 4(-2) = -1$
You must multiply the O.S. of O by the number of O molecules in the molecule (in this case 4).
Solve the equation.
$x - 8 = -1$
So,
$x = +7$
Therefore, the O.S. of Mn is (VII).

Getting to Know the Topic:

Now, try a few on your own

(i) $\underline{C}Cl_4$

(ii) $K_2\underline{Cr}_2O_7$

(iii) $K\underline{Cl}O_3$

(iv) $\underline{C}N^-$

(v) $\underline{P}_2O_7^{4-}$

(vi) $Na_2\underline{S}_4O_6$

(vii) $Mg_3\underline{N}_2$

Solution

(i) CCl_4
$x + 4 (-1) = 0 \quad x = + 4$
O.S. of C is (IV).

(ii) $K_2Cr_2O_7$
$2 (+1) + 2x + 7 (-2) = 0; x = +6$
O.S. of Cr is (VI).

(iii) $KClO_3$
$1 (+1) + x + 3 (-2) = 0; x = +5$
O.S. of Cl is (V).

(iv) CN^-
$x + 1(-3) = -1; \qquad x = +2$
O.S. of C is (II).

(v) $P_2O_7^{4-}$
$2x + 7(-2) = -4; \quad x = +5$
O.S. of P is (V).

(vi) $Na_2S_4O_6$
$2 (+1) + 4x + 6(-2) = 0; x = + 2.5$
O.S. of S is (+2.5).
Oxidation number (state) can be a fraction. Note that it is an apparent charge on the atom.

(vii) Mg_3N_2
$3(+2) + 2x = 0; \quad x = -3$
O.S. of N is (-III).

GAMSAT Style Question

Question (1-3)

Oxidation-reduction (redox) reactions involve the transfer of electrons from one atom to another resulting in the oxidation of one molecule and the reduction of another within a reaction. Oxidation can be defined as the loss of electrons by an atom. Consider the following redox reaction:

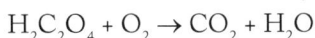

$$H_2C_2O_4 + O_2 \rightarrow CO_2 + H_2O$$

1. In this reaction, what happens to the oxidation state of C?
   A. It is oxidized by a value of 1/2
   B. It is oxidized by a value of 1
   C. It is reduced by a value of 1
   D. It does not change

2. Given the following molecules
   A. $CH_2=CH_2$
   B. CO_2
   C. $CH\equiv CH$
   D. CH_3CH_3

   List these compounds in order of increasing oxidation state of carbon
   A. $CH_3CH_3 < CO_2 < CH\equiv CH < CH_2=CH_2$
   B. $CH\equiv CH < CH_3CH_3 < CH_2=CH_2 < CO_2$
   C. $CO_2 < CH_3CH_3 < CH_2=CH_2 < CH\equiv CH$
   D. $CH_3CH_3 < CH_2=CH_2 < CH\equiv CH < CO_2$

3. Consider the following reaction involving the transformation of ethanol to acetic acid

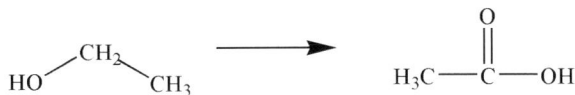

Which of the following statements is true?

A. Ethanol is being reduced because the oxidation state of C has increased with the addition of the oxygen

B. Ethanol is being reduced because the oxidation state of C has decreased with the addition of the oxygen

C. Ethanol is being oxidized because the oxidation state of C has increased with the addition of the oxygen

D. Ethanol is being oxidized because the oxidation state of C has decreased with the addition of the oxygen

Solution

Question 1

STEP 1 = > What do you need to determine to solve the problem?
You need to find the oxidation state of carbon in the reactants and in the products of the reaction to determine how it changes within the reaction.

STEP 2 = > What relevant data provided in this problem is necessary in order to answer the question?
You are provided with the chemical reaction equation. This will allow you to calculate the O.S. of carbon. Recall, the O.S. of O in most molecules is -2, and that of H in all molecules except metallic hydrides is $+1$.

STEP 3 = > Use the relevant data to solve the question
To solve this problem, you must first determine the O.S. state of C in $H_2C_2O_4$ and CO_2.
For $H_2C_2O_4$
$2(+1) + 2x + 4(-2) = 0$
$x = +3$, so the oxidation state for C is $+3$.

For CO_2
$x + 2(-2) = 0$
$x = +4$, so the oxidation state for C is $+4$.

Thus, you can see that the O.S. has increased by a value of 1 (from $+3$ to $+4$) in the course of the reaction. Now, you need to recall that an increase in oxidation state is called an oxidation and a lowering of oxidation state is a reduction (Hint: reducing the price of something makes it lower, which is analogous to reducing the oxidation state of a molecule). Therefore the correct answer is B.

Question 2

STEP 1 = > What do you need to determine to solve the problem?

You need to determine the oxidation state of C in the different compounds and list them in order of increasing oxidation state.

STEP 2 = > What relevant data provided in this problem is necessary in order to answer the question?

You are provided with the chemical structures of the different molecules. This will allow you to calculate the O.S. of carbon. Recall, the O.S. of O in most molecules is –2, and that of H in all molecules except metallic hydrides is +1. You are also told that oxidation is the loss of electrons by an atom.

STEP 3 = > Use the relevant data to solve the question

So, now, you simply calculate the O.S. of each compound

$CH_2=CH_2$

$2x + 4(+1) = 0$

$x = -2$

CO_2

$x + 2(-2) = 0$

$x = 4$

$CH\equiv CH$

$2x + 2(+1) = 0$

$x = -1$

CH_3CH_3

$2x + 6(+1) = 0$

$x = -3$

Remember, oxidation is the loss of electrons by an atom, which means that compound with the lowest oxidation state will have the most negative charge, and that with the highest oxidation state will have the most positive charge.

So, the correct order is D. CH_3CH_3 < $CH_2=CH_2$ < $CH\equiv CH$ < CO_2

Question 3

STEP 1 = > What do you need to determine to solve the problem?

You need to determine what has happened to the oxidation state of C in the course of the reaction, and then determine the correct statement.

STEP 2 = > What relevant data provided in this problem is necessary in order to answer the question?

You are provided with the chemical reaction showing the transformation of ethanol to acetic acid. Given the chemical structure of both molecules, you can calculate the O.S. of carbon. Recall, the O.S. of O in most molecules is –2, and that of H in all molecules except metallic hydrides is +1. You are also told that oxidation is the loss of electrons.

STEP 3 = > Use the relevant data to solve the question

The O.S. of ethanol is

C_2H_5OH

$2x + 6(+1) + 1(-2) = 0$

$x = -2$

The O.S. of acetic acid

CH_3COOH

$2x + 2(-2) + 4(+1) = 0$

$x = 0$

So, you can see that the oxidation state has increased during the transformation. Remember, since oxidation can be defined as a loss of electrons, when a substance is oxidized, that means the O.S. becomes more positive. So, the correct answer is C.

Chapter 3: **Enthalpy and Internal Energy**

Key Concepts: Enthalpy

Enthalpy is a measure of heat in the system. Scientists figure out the mass of a substance when it is under a constant pressure. Once they have figured out the mass, they measure the internal energy of the system. All together, that energy is the enthalpy. The formula "$\Delta H = \Delta E + P \Delta V$ " defines the enthalpy of a system, where ΔH is the enthalpy value, ΔE is the amount of internal energy, and P and ΔV are the Pressure and Volume of the system. The internal energy is related to the work done by the system (w) and the energy transfer across the system (q). Therefore, $\Delta E = q+w$. Any mechanical work must change the volume (something must move); under normal conditions where the pressure stays constant, $w = -p\Delta V$.

- When $\Delta H > 0$, the reaction absorbs heat and is therefore endothermic
- When $\Delta H < 0$, the reaction lets off heat and is therefore exothermic
- When $w > 0$, the system does external work
- When $w < 0$, work is done on the system
- When $q > 0$, the system absorbs heat
- When $q < 0$, the system gives off heat

Note: Memorize these points.

When a chemical reaction occurs in an open container, the energy gained or lost is in the form of heat, almost no work is done. When a chemical reaction occurs and the system absorbs heat, the process is endothermic and when the chemical reaction produces heat, it is exothermic. Enthalpy is not measured directly, but rather the heat added or lost by the system or the change in enthalpy (ΔH). Because the change in enthalpy is described by the final and initial enthalpies, the ΔH for a chemical reaction can be described by comparing the enthalpies of the products and the reactants. For example,

$$\Delta H = H(products) - H(reactants)$$

The resulting change in enthalpy is called the enthalpy of reaction (ΔH_{rxn}). Many times you will see the ΔH_{rxn} along with balanced chemical equations (thermochemical equation) for the reaction.

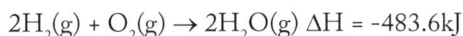

$$2H_2(g) + O_2(g) \rightarrow 2H_2O(g) \; \Delta H = -483.6kJ$$

In this case, since ΔH is negative the reaction is releasing heat and therefore exothermic.

—>*Quick Facts:* Properties of Enthalpy

- Enthalpy is an extensive property
    - o The magnitude of ΔH depends on the amounts of reactants consumed
    - o Doubling the reactants, doubles the amount of enthalpy
- Reversing a chemical reaction results in the same magnitude but opposite sign
- The enthalpy change for a reaction depends on the state of the reactants and products

Illustrative Questions

1. Given that the heat of fusion of ice is 333 J/g and the heat of vaporization of water is 2257 J/g. Calculate the change in enthalpy, ΔH, for the following processes.

$H_2O(s) \rightarrow H_2O(l)$

$H_2O(l) \rightarrow H_2O(g)$

2. Calculate the change in enthalpy, ΔH, for the following reaction:

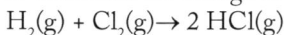

$H_2(g) + Cl_2(g) \rightarrow 2\ HCl(g)$

Given single bond energies for the H-H and Cl-Cl bonds are +436 kJ/mol and + 243 kJ/mol respectively. For H-Cl it is 431 kJ/mol.

Solution

1. First, you must determine the m.w. of water, which are 18.02 g/mol

For fusion

$\Delta H = 18.02\ g \times 333\ J/g$

$\Delta H = 6.00 \times 10^3\ J = 6.00\ kJ$

For vaporization

$\Delta H = 18.02\ g \times 2257\ J/g$

$\Delta H = 4.07 \times 10^4\ J = 40.7\ kJ$

2. Think of how the reaction proceeds, first the molecules will break down and then they will combine in a second step to form HCl, so you need to calculate both ΔH's for the two steps. In this first step, 1 mole of H_2 and Cl_2 is broken down as follows:

$H_2(g) \rightarrow 2\ H(g)$

$Cl_2(g) \rightarrow 2\ Cl(g)$

So $\Delta H_1 = (436 + 243) = 679$ kJ/mol

In the second step, the two combined to make 2 moles of HCl as follows:

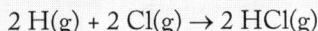

$2 H(g) + 2 Cl(g) \rightarrow 2 HCl(g)$
So $\Delta H_2 = -2(431) = -862$ kJ/mol
So add up the ΔH's to calculate the overall change in enthalpy.

$\Delta H = 679 + (-862) = -183$ kJ/mol

Getting to Know the Topic:

Questions 1–8

The relation between the enthalpy and the internal energy is given by the equation,
$\Delta H = \Delta E + P \Delta V$,
Where ΔH = change in enthalpy
And ΔE = change in internal energy
For a reaction involving gaseous components at constant T and P, we have
$\Delta V = \Delta n_g RT/P$

1. For which of the following reactions does ΔH equal the internal energy change?
   A. $2Na(s) + 2H_2O(1) \rightarrow 2NaOH(aq) + H_2(g)$
   B. $NaCl(aq) + AgNO_3(aq) \rightarrow NaNO_3(aq) + AgCl(s)$
   C. $2H_2(g) + O_2(g) \rightarrow 2H_2O(1)$
   D. $2C(s) + O_2(g) \rightarrow 2CO(g)$

2. The value of $\Delta H - \Delta E$ for the following reaction at a temperature T is
   $C_4H_{10}(g) + 13/2 O_2(g) \rightarrow 4CO_2(g) + 5H_2O(1)$
   A. -3/2 RT
   B. -5/2 RT
   C. -1/2 RT
   D. -7/2 RT

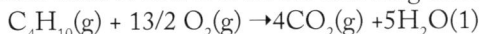

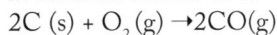

3. The difference between the enthalpy and the internal energy at constant pressure and at constant volume at 27° C for the following reaction is
   $2C(s) + O_2(g) \rightarrow 2CO(g)$
   $(R = 8.3 \text{ J mol}^{-1} \text{ K}^{-1})$
   A. 2490 kJ mol^{-1}
   B. -2490 J mol^{-1}
   C. +1.25 kJ mol^{-1}
   D. 2.490 kJ mol^{-1}

4. For the vaporization of water, which of the following statements is CORRECT?

    A. $\Delta H = \Delta E$

    B. $\Delta H > \Delta E$

    C. $\Delta H < \Delta E$

    D. $\Delta H = \Delta E + \Delta n_g RT$

5. Calculate the internal energy change for the following reaction at 298K?

$(R = 8.0 \text{ J mol}^{-1} \text{ K}^{-1})$
$C(s) + 2H_2(g) \rightarrow CH_4(g) \; \Delta H = -74 \text{ kJ mol}^{-1}$

    A. -76.40 kJ mol^{-1}

    B. +2310 kJ mol^{-1}

    C. -71.60 kJ mol^{-1}

    D. -2458 kJ mol^{-1}

6. For a given reaction at constant T and P, the enthalpy change and the internal energy change at 298 K are -11 K cal/mol and -10.4 K cal/mol respectively. Which of the following statements is true:
$(R = 2 \text{ cal mol}^{-1} \text{ K}^{-1})$

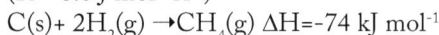

    A. Equal number of moles of gaseous species are present on both sides of the reaction

    B. There are a greater number of moles of gaseous products than the number of moles of gaseous reactions

    C. Number of moles of gaseous reactants equals to twice the number of moles of gaseous products

    D. Number of moles of gaseous products is less than the number of moles of gaseous reactants

7. In all the following reactants, heat at constant pressure is greater than the heat at constant volume EXCEPT

    A. $CH_4(g) + 2O_2(g) \rightarrow CO_2(g) + 2H_2O(l)$

    B. $2Na(s) + 2HCl(aq) \rightarrow 2NaCl(s) + H_2(g)$

    C. $NH_3(g) \rightarrow 1/2 \, N_2(g) + 3/2 \, H_2(g)$

    D. $H_2(g) + I_2(g) \rightarrow 2HI(g)$

8. An adiabatic process is one in which there is no transfer of heat across the boundary between system and surroundings. For such a process

A. ΔV=0

B. q=w

C. ΔE=w

D. ΔE=q

Question 9–12

It's also given that ΔE = q+w.
Useful conversions:
(1 atm = 101325 Pa)
(1 Pa m^3 = 1 kJ)

9. A gas is compressed by a constant external pressure of 1.50 atm from 8.00 to 2.00 L in volume, 100kJ of heat is absorbed in the process. What is ΔE for the gas?

A. -812kJ

B. +812kJ

C. +912kJ

D. 1012kJ

10. A gas expands against a constant external pressure of 2.00 atm from an initial volume of 1.50 L to a final volume of 3.50 L. The container is well insulated so that no heat enters or leaves the system. Calculate the change in internal energy ΔE of the gas in kilojoules.

A. -405

B. +405

C. 4.05

D. 25.3

11. Which of the following is an exothermic process?

A. Melting ice

B. Splitting a gas molecule

C. Rusting iron

D. Sublimation of dry ice

12. Which of the following is an endothermic process?

    A. Mixing water with a strong acid

    B. Evaporation of water

    C. Forming ion pairs

    D. Burning sugar

Questions 13–15

The standard enthalpy of formation is the amount of heat absorbed at constant pressure when 1 mole of a compound is formed from its elements in their standard state.

13. For which of the following equations is the enthalpy change at 298 K and 1 atm equal to $\Delta H°f (CH_3OH)$ (l)?

    A. $C(s) + 4H(g) + O(g) \rightarrow CH_3OH(l)$

    B. $C(s) + H_2O(g) + H_2(g) \rightarrow CH_3OH(l)$

    C. $C(s) + 2H_2(g) + 1/2\ O_2(g) \rightarrow CH_3OH(1)$

    D. $C(s) + 2H_2\ (g) + 1/2\ O_2(l) \rightarrow CH_3OH(l)$

14. In which of the following reactions at 298 K and 1 atm enthalpy change is equal to $\Delta H°f(CO_2)$ (g)?

    A. $CH_4\ (g) + 2O_2(g) \rightarrow CO_2(g) + 2H_2O(l)$

    B. $C(g) + O_2(g) \rightarrow CO_2(g)$

    C. $CO(s) + 1/2O_2(g) \rightarrow CO_2(g)$

    D. $CO(g) + 1/2O_2(g) \rightarrow CO_2(g)$

15. Which of the following equations correctly represent the standard heat of formation ($\Delta H°$ of methane)

    A. $C\ (diamond) + 4H\ (g) \rightarrow CH_4\ (g)$

    B. $C\ (graphite) + 2H_2\ (g) \rightarrow CH_4\ (g)$

    C. $C\ (graphite) + 4H\ (g) \rightarrow CH_4\ (g)$

    D. $C\ (diamond) + 2H_2\ (g) \rightarrow CH_4\ (g)$

Question 16–17

The standard enthalpy of a reaction is defined as the difference between the reaction enthalpies of formation of the products and the standard enthalpies for the formation of reactants.

16. The standard enthalpies of formation for carbon dioxide and formic acid are -393.7 kJ mol $^{-1}$ and -409.2 kJ mol $^{-1}$ respectively. What is the enthalpy change in kJ mol^{-1}, for the reaction?

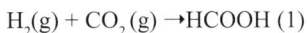

$H_2(g) + CO_2(g) \rightarrow HCOOH (l)$

    A. -802.9
    B. +802.9
    C. -15.5
    D. +15.5

17. From the data below, the value of $\Delta H°$ in kJ for the reaction:

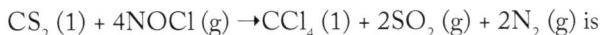

$CS_2 (l) + 4NOCl (g) \rightarrow CCl_4 (l) + 2SO_2 (g) + 2N_2 (g)$ is

$\Delta H°f$ (kJ mol^{-1})	88	53	-139	-296
Substance	$CS_2(l)$	$NOCl(g)$	$CCl_4(l)$	$SO_2(g)$

    A. -1031
    B. -731
    C. -431
    D. +431

Solution

Question 1

STEP 1 = > What do you need to determine to solve the problem?
We have to determine among the given choices, in which equation ΔH equals the internal energy change.

STEP 2 = > What relevant data provided in this problem is necessary in order to answer the question?
We have been given the basic equation that relates the parameters.

STEP 3 = > Use the relevant data to solve the question
$\Delta H = \Delta E + P\Delta V$
For a reaction involving gaseous components at constant T and P, we have
$\Delta V = \Delta n_g RT/P$
$\therefore \ \Delta H = \Delta E + P\Delta n_g RT/P$
or $\Delta H - \Delta E = \Delta n_g RT$

$\Delta H = \Delta E$ only when $\Delta n_g = 0$. Only for reaction B, $\Delta n_g = 0$ because there is no gaseous component involved. The answer is B.

Question 2

$\Delta n_g = 4 - (1 + 13/2) = -7/2$
$\Delta H = \Delta E + - 7/2 \ RT$
or $\Delta H - \Delta E = -7/2 \ RT$ which is answer D.

Question 3

$\Delta n_g = 2 - 1 = 1$
$\Delta H - \Delta E = \Delta n_g RT = RT = 8.3 \ J \ mol^{-1} \ k^{-1} \times 300 \ k$
$\Delta H - \Delta E = 2490 \ J \ mol^{-1} = 2.490 \ kJ \ mol^{-1}$
The answer is D.

Question 4

The vapourization of water is
$H_2O(1) \rightarrow H_2O \ (g)$
in which $\Delta n_g = 1$
Therefore $\Delta H = \Delta E + RT$
and ΔH will be greater than ΔE ($\Delta n_g > 0$)
The answer is B.

Question 5

$\Delta n_g = 1 - 2 = -1$

$\Delta H = -74$ kJ mol^{-1}

$\Delta E = \Delta H - \Delta n_g RT$

$= -74$ kJ mol^{-1} $- (-1) \times 0.008$ kJ k^{-1} mol$^{-1} \times 298$ K

$= -71.6$ kJ mol^{-1} which is answer C.

Question 6

In this case, the question tells you that $\Delta H = -11$ K cal/mol and $\Delta E = -10.4$ K cal/mol, so $\Delta H < \Delta E$. Use the following equation $\Delta H = \Delta E + P\Delta n_g RT/P$. Since you are told that the reaction is done at constant T and P, you know that $\Delta H = \Delta E + \Delta n_g RT$. You know that R is a constant, and T must be greater than 0 since T must be in Kelvin and is constant. This means that the only unknown variable is Δn_g. So, since $\Delta H < \Delta E$, and $\Delta H = \Delta E + \Delta n_g RT$, and RT are positive, this means that Δn_g must be <0. In order for $\Delta n_g < 0$ the number of moles of gaseous products must be less than the number of moles of gaseous reactants. The correct answer is D.

Question 7

ΔH will be greater than ΔE (heat at constant volume) only when $\Delta n_g > 0$ (more gaseous products than gaseous reactants). This occurs only in answer A. Therefore in A, ΔH will not be greater than ΔE.

Question 8

In adiabatic process, there is no exchange of heat between the system and the surrounding. i.e. q = 0

$\therefore$ from 1st law of thermodynamic

$\Delta E = q + w$; q = 0

$\Delta E = w$, the answer is C.

Question 9

q = + 100 kJ

Any mechanical work must change the volume (something must move); under normal conditions where the pressure stays constant, $w = p\Delta V$

Therefore, $w = p\Delta V = 1.50$ atm $(8.00$ L$- 2.00$L$) = 1.50 \times 6$ L atm = 9 L atm. Now, note that the possible answers are in units of kilojoules, and w is in units of L atm. Therefore, a conversion must be done to get w is the proper units. The question states that 1 atm = 101325 Pa and that 1 Pa m^3 = 1 kJ. It is very important that you simply commit to memory that 1 L = 1×10^{-3}m^3. So you must convert 9 atm m^3 to J.

$(9 \times 10^{-3}$ atm m$^3) \times (101325$ Pa$/$ 1 atm$) \times (1$k J$/1$Pa m$^3) = 911925$ J

w = 912 kJ

$\Delta E = q + w = 100 + 912 = +1012$ kJ

The answer is D.

Question 10

Since no heat is gained or lost, q = 0

$\Delta E = w = p\Delta V = 2$ atm $\times$ (1.5 L - 3.5 L) = -4 atm L. Again, a conversion is needed.

(-4 atm m^3)$\times$(101325 Pa/ 1 atm)$\times$(1J/1Pa m^3) = -405300 J = -405 kJ

$\Delta E = -405$ kJ, the answer is A.

Question 11

The correct answer is C. An exothermic process is one which gives off heat. In order to melt an ice cube, the ice absorbs heat from its surroundings. In order to split apart gas molecules, heat is required to break the bond. Finally, the sublimation of dry ice which is the conversion from the solid phase into the gas phase is similar to melting ice, the dry ice must take in heat to sublimate. The formation of rust is a chemical reaction in which heat is given off. Even if you did not know this, you could use the process of elimination.

Question 12

The correct answer is B. An endothermic process is one which heat is absorbed. The evaporation of water involves the conversion of a liquid to gas. To accomplish this, heat must be absorbed by the water for it to evaporate.

Question 13

The standard enthalpy of formation is the amount of heat absorbed at constant pressure when 1 mole of a compound is formed from its elements in their standard state. Therefore $\Delta H = \Delta H°_f$

For the formation of 1 mole of $CH_3OH(l)$, the only equation where the elements are in their standard state is equation C. Remember, the question states that the reaction is at 1 atm and 298 K, elements MUST be in their standard state under these conditions.

Question 14

The first reaction involves more than one product. As a result, the enthalpy change cannot be $\Delta H°_f (CO_2)(g)$. In the second and third reaction, the formation of $CO_2(g)$ is not from the standard elements. Therefore, the answer is D. This involves the formation of 1 mole of CO_2 from its elements in their standard state.

Question 15

At 298 K and 1 atm, the standard state of carbon is graphite. $\Delta H°_f (CH_4)$ is the enthalpy change when 1 mole of CH_4 is formed from its elements H_2 (g) and C (graphite) in their standard state. That is present only in equation B.

Question 16

$\Delta H^\circ_r = \Delta H^\circ_f HCOOH (1) - [\Delta H^\circ_f H_2(g) + \Delta H^\circ_r CO_2(g)]$
=409.2 – (0-393.7)
= -409.2 + 393.7 = -15.5 kJ mol^{-1}
The answer is C.

Question 17

$\Delta H^\circ_f (N_2)_g = 0$
$\Delta H^\circ = [-139 + 2 \times (-296)] - [88 + 4(53)]$
    = (-139 -592)-(300)
    = -1031 kJ mol^{-1} which is answer A.

GAMSAT Style Questions

Question 1

1. ΔH of three different reactions are given below.

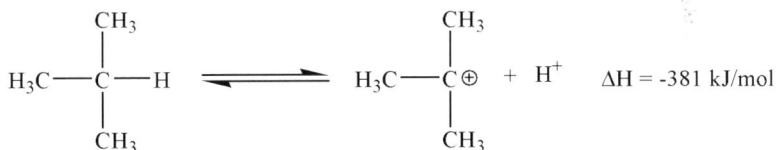

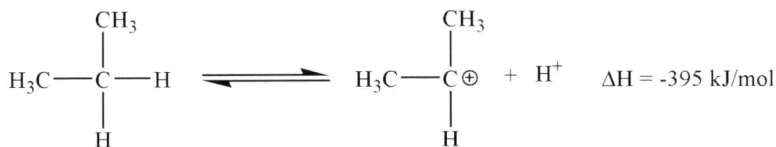

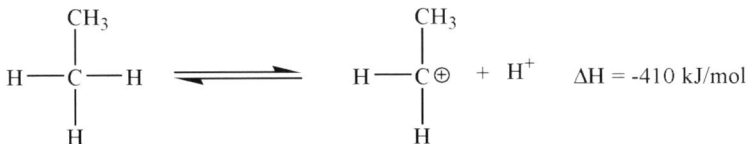

$$(CH_3)_3CH \rightleftharpoons (CH_3)_3C^{\oplus} + H^+ \qquad \Delta H = -381 \text{ kJ/mol}$$

$$(CH_3)_2CH_2 \rightleftharpoons (CH_3)_2CH^{\oplus} + H^+ \qquad \Delta H = -395 \text{ kJ/mol}$$

$$CH_3CH_3 \rightleftharpoons CH_3CH_2^{\oplus} + H^+ \qquad \Delta H = -410 \text{ kJ/mol}$$

From the above data, we can infer that the stability of the given free radicals increases in the following order,

A.

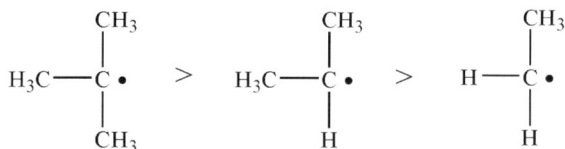

B.

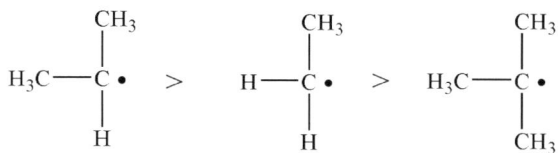

C.

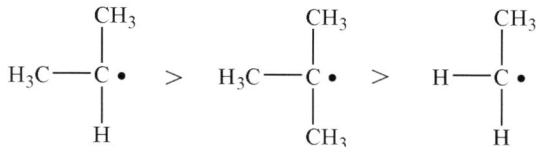

D. It's impossible to gauge stability from the above data.

Questions 2–3

Enthalpy is related to the internal energy, pressure and volume of a system by the following equation: $\Delta H = \Delta E + \Delta(PV)$. The simplest calculation of ΔH occurs in a constant pressure process in a closed system. For this case, ΔH is simply equal to the amount of heat transferred in the process denoted by q. The first law of thermodynamics tells us that the change internal energy of the system is equal to the heat transferred plus the amount of work done or $\Delta E = q + w$.

2. Given a simple constant pressure closed system, which of the following statements are true?

    A. ΔE will be equal to q

    B. ΔE will be equal to w

    C. q and w will be equal

    D. None of the above

3. For a system that is insulated, no heat is transferred to or from the system. Given the above equations, what equation defines the ΔH for this type of system?

    A. $\Delta H = \Delta E$

    B. $\Delta H = q + w$

    C. $\Delta H = w + \Delta E$

    D. $\Delta H = w + \Delta(PV)$

Questions 4-5

4. The enthalpy of a reaction is defined as the difference between the enthalpies of formation of the products and the enthalpies for the formation of reactants. The standard state enthalpy change for the combustion of methane at 298K is −890.4 kJ mol^{-1}, resulting in the formation of water as one of the products. Find the enthalpy of the reaction at 298K given the following unbalanced reaction.

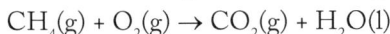

$$CH_4(g) + O_2(g) \rightarrow CO_2(g) + H_2O(l)$$

At 298K

$\Delta H_f (CO_2(g)) = -393.5$ kJ mol^{-1}

$\Delta H_f (H_2O(l)) = -285.8$ kJ mol^{-1}

$\Delta H_f (O_2(g)) = 0$ kJ mol^{-1}

    A. 74.4 kJ mol^{-1}

    B. -74.7 kJ mol^{-1}

    C. 211.1 kJ mol^{-1}

    D. -211.1 kJ mol^{-1}

5. The spontaneity of a reaction involves two variables, enthalpy and entropy. Enthalpy (H) is defined as the amount of heat absorbed by a system at constant pressure. Entropy (S) is a measure of the amount of disorder or randomness in a system. The relationship between reaction spontaneity, entropy and enthalpy is given by the Gibbs free energy function:

$$\Delta G = \Delta H - T\,\Delta S$$

Given a reaction at constant temperature and pressure, what is true about ΔG at equilibrium?

    A. ΔG is negative

    B. ΔG is positive

    C. ΔG is 0

    D. The answer cannot be determined from the provided information

Solution

Question 1

STEP 1 = > What do you need to determine to solve the problem?
The stability of the free radicals in the three different equations must be determined.

STEP 2 = > What relevant data provided in this problem is necessary in order to answer the question?
Three dissociation reactions have been provided along with the ΔH for each reaction. The ΔH becomes more negative with decreasing numbers of methyl side groups.

STEP 3 = > Use the relevant data to solve the question
From the given data it can be inferred that the bond-breaking reaction become more stable as the number of alkyl groups increases. This is indicated by the fact that it takes *less energy* to break a C—H bond as the number of alkyl groups on the carbon atom that contains this bond increases. Hence the answer is A.

Question 2

STEP 1 = > What do you need to determine to solve the problem?
You need to find the correct statement from those provided.

STEP 2 = > What relevant data provided in this problem is necessary in order to answer the question?
You have been provided equations relating internal energy ΔE, enthalpy ΔH, heat q, and work w. You are also told that it is a closed, constant pressure system.

STEP 3 = > Use the relevant data to solve the question
Since you have a closed constant pressure system, you know that there will be no change in pressure or volume thus $\Delta H = \Delta E$. You are also told in the problem, that ΔH is equal to q for this type of system. Therefore, the correct answer is A.

Question 3

STEP 1 = > What do you need to determine to solve the problem?
You need to determine which equation describes the ΔH for an insulated system.

STEP 2 = > What relevant data provided in this problem is necessary in order to answer the question?
You have been provided equations relating internal energy ΔE, enthalpy ΔH, heat q, and work w. You are also told that this is an insulated system so there is no heat transfer.

STEP 3 = > Use the relevant data to solve the question
With no heat transfer q = 0. Therefore, $\Delta E = w$.
Subsequently, $\Delta H = \Delta E + \Delta(PV) = w + \Delta(PV)$. The answer is D.

Question 4

STEP 1 = > What do you need to determine to solve the problem?
You need to calculate the enthalpy of the reaction.

STEP 2 = > What relevant data provided in this problem is necessary in order to answer the question?
You are provided with an UNBALANCED chemical reaction and the heats of formation for the different reactants and products. You are also told that the enthalpy of the reactions is equal to the difference between the enthalpies of formation of the products and the enthalpies for the formation of reactants.

STEP 3 = > Use the relevant data to solve the question
First you need to balance the reaction:

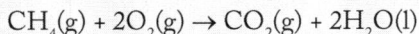

$$CH_4(g) + 2O_2(g) \rightarrow CO_2(g) + 2H_2O(l)$$

Next, you need to add up the ΔH_f for the products and the reactants.

ΔH_fproducts = 1(-393.5) + 2(-285.8) = -965.1
ΔH_freactants = 1(-890.4) + 2(0) = -890.4
ΔH_fproducts - ΔH_freactants = ΔH = -74.7 kJ mol^{-1}
The answer is B.

Question 5

STEP 1 = > What do you need to determine to solve the problem?
You need to determine what ΔG would be at equilibrium.

STEP 2 = > What relevant data provided in this problem is necessary in order to answer the question?
You are provided the equation relating ΔG to ΔH, T and ΔS. You are also told that ΔG is related to the spontaneity of the system, thus it dictates whether the reaction will proceed forward.

STEP 3 = > Use the relevant data to solve the question
The answer is C. This is a fairly simple concept that may seem more difficult due to the large amount of information provided in the question. In reality, you do not need the equation given you simply need to grasp the concept of ΔG. In order for a reaction to proceed, ΔG must be negative. Since ΔG is related to the progression of the reaction, and at equilibrium, the reaction proceeds in neither direction, ΔG will be zero.

Chapter 4: **Behaviour of Gases**

Key Concepts: Behaviour of Gases

Boyle's Law (*Relation between the volume and pressure of a gas*)

"The volume of a given mass of a dry gas is inversely proportional to the pressure, if the temperature remains constant," i.e. $V \propto \frac{1}{P}$, or PV = constant

If the volume of a given mass of a gas is V_1 under pressure P_1 and changes to V_2 under pressure P_2, at constant temperature, then $P_1 \times V_1 = P_2 \times V_2$

Let's look at a practical example of this law. Imagine you have a balloon that measures 50cm³ at the surface of the ocean. At sea level, the balloon is currently under 1 atm of pressure. Now, if we push the balloon underwater to a depth of 10 meters, it is now subjected to 2 atm of pressure (one from the air at the surface and one from the water). Since there is now twice the pressure, the volume of the balloon will decrease by 1/2. Thus, in 10 meters of water, the balloon will occupy only 25 cm³. By bringing the balloon back to the surface, it returns to its original size. This occurs because the air inside the balloon is compressed when it is taken under water and then expands when the balloon is taken back to the surface.

Charle's Law (*Relation between the volume and temperature of a gas*)

" The volume of a dry gas is directly proportional to the temperature, if the pressure remains constant," i.e. $\frac{V}{T}$ = constant

If the volume of a given mass of gas is V_1 at temperature T_1 and changes to V_2 at temperature T_2, at a constant pressure, then $\frac{V_1}{T_1} = \frac{V_2}{T_2}$

Another way to make the balloon smaller other than increasing the pressure exerted on the balloon is to change the temperature. If you take the same balloon was mentioned above and put it into the freezer, it will shrink. If you heat up the same balloon, it will expand. What happens here is that by increasing the temperature, molecular motion of the gas molecules inside the balloon increases. As the gas molecules move faster, they hit the sides of the balloon more often causing expansion. Cooling the gas has the opposite effect, molecular motion slows down, the number of collisions decreases, and the balloon shrinks. A real life example of this law is a hot air balloon. As the air in the balloon is heated, it expands and fills.

Gay-Lussac's Law

"The pressure of a dry gas is directly proportional to the temperature, if the volume remains constant," i.e. $\frac{P}{T}$ = constant

If the pressure of a given mass of gas is P_1 at temperature T_1 and changes to P_2 at temperature T_2, at a constant volume, then $\frac{P_1}{T_1} = \frac{P_2}{T_2}$

So, now instead of a balloon, we have a rigid container that is unable to increase or decrease in size. For instance, a gas canister or spray can. If you increase the temperature, similar to described above, molecular motion increases. But now, instead of a subsequent expansion of the container, because the container is rigid, the increase in molecules hitting the sides of the container results in an increase in pressure. This can be dangerous if the container is unable to accommodate the increase in pressure and an explosion of the container can result.

The Combined Gas law

Combining, Boyle's law, Charles' law, and Gay-Lussac's Law, $V \propto \frac{T}{P}$, or

$\frac{PV}{T}$ = constant

The combined gas law deals with gas systems where the quantity of gas is kept constant.

This relation is called the combined gas equation, and the relation becomes:

$$\frac{P_1 \times V_1}{T_1} = \frac{P_2 \times V_2}{T_2} \quad \text{or}$$

$$V_2 = \frac{P_1 \times V_1}{T_1} \times \frac{T_2}{P_2}$$

This law combines the previous three laws and describes the relationship between pressure, volume, and temperature. It can be used to solve any Boyle's law, Charles' law, or Gay-Lussac's law problems, just omit the variable that is held constant.

Avogadro's law

At a constant temperature and pressure, the volume of a gas is directly proportional to the number of moles of that gas; $\frac{V}{n}$ = constant

This relationship becomes

$$\frac{V_1}{n_1} = \frac{V_2}{n_2}$$

What this says is that if the amount of gas in a container is increased, the volume increases. If the amount of gas in a container is decreased, the volume decreases.

Suppose the amount is increased. This means there are more gas molecules and this will increase the number of impacts on the container walls. This means the gas pressure inside the container will increase (for an instant), becoming greater than the pressure on the outside of the walls. This causes the walls to move outward. Since there is more wall space the impacts will lessen and the pressure will return to its original value.

Two important corollaries to this law are

(1) Molecular weight = 22.4 × vapour density.

(2) One mole (i.e. one gram molecular weight) of any gas occupies 22.4 litres at **N.T.P.**

The volume 22.4 litres is known as the gram molecular volume (**G. M. V.**).

Standard Conditions

Standard temperature and pressure (**STP**) is defined at 0°C (273 K) and 1 atm of pressure. These conditions are important for measurements and documentation of chemical and physical properties and refer to nominal conditions in the atmosphere at sea level.

Another set of conditions is normal temperature and pressure (**NTP**). This is defined at 20°C and 1 atm and is common for testing and documentation of fan capacities.

The molar volume is the volume occupied by a mole of a substance at STP. According to Avogadro's law, at a given temperature and pressure a given volume of any gas contains the same number of molecules. Thus, at STP 1 mole of gas occupies 22.4 litres. This value is known as the gram molecular volume (**GMV**) of a gas.

Avogadro's Number.

The number of molecules present in one gram-molecular weight of any gas is the same. This number is called Avogadro's number or Avogadro's constant. It is equal to 6.023×10^{23}. This is the number of molecules present in a mole of any substance.

Knowing the molecular weight of a substance and Avogadro's number, the weight in grams of one single molecule can be calculated. For example, the molecular weight of oxygen is 32 (gram

molecular weight = 32 grams), hence the weight of 1 molecule of oxygen $= \dfrac{32}{6.023 \times 10^{23}}$

$= 5.314 \times 10^{-23}$ grams

Equation of Ideal Gas

The three historically important gas laws derived relationships between two physical properties of a gas, while keeping other properties constant: Boyle's law, Charles' law, and Avogadro's law. The three relationships can be combined to make a more general gas law.

$$V \propto \frac{nT}{P}$$

If the fixed mass of gas is 1 mole, every gas will occupy the same volume at a given. Hence, for 1 mole of any gas, independent of its nature, $\dfrac{PV}{T}$ has the same value, R.

That is, $\dfrac{PV}{T} = R$ or $PV = n\,RT$

For n gram molecules, $PV = nRT$

       V is the volume occupied by 1 gram molecule of the gas,

       P is the pressure exerted by the gas,

       T is the temperature in A or K,

       n is the number of gram molecules of the gas.

The equation $PV = n\,RT$ is the ideal gas equation.

If g is the weight of the gas and M is its molecular weight, $n = \dfrac{g}{M}$; $\dfrac{M}{g} PV = RT$

A few important points should be noted when using the ideal gas equation.

- An "ideal gas" is one whose physical behaviour is accurately described by the ideal-gas equation
- The constant R is called the gas constant
  - The value and units of R depend on the units used in determining P, V, n and T
  - Temperature, T, must always be expressed on an absolute-temperature scale (K)
  - The quantity of gas, n, is normally expressed in *moles*
  - The units chosen for pressure and volume are typically *atmospheres* (*atm*) and *liters* (*l*), however, other units may be chosen
  - PV can have the units of energy

van der Waals Gas Law (deviations from the ideal gas law)

The van der Waals equation is an attempt to improve the ideal gas law by including repulsive and attractive molecular interactions and the non-zero volume taken up by the molecules themselves. The equation is

$$P = \frac{nRT}{(V-nb)} - a(\frac{n}{V})^2$$

In the ideal gas law, the gas particles are assumed not to interact and to have no size. In the van der Waals equation, the repulsive interactions and non-zero size of the molecules are taken into account by supposing that the molecules are only free to move in a volume *V-nb* where nb is approximately the volume occupied by the molecules themselves.

The pressure exerted by the gas on the walls of the container is related to the number and frequency of the collisions with the wall. These are both reduced by attractive forces between the molecules and this is included in the $-a(\frac{n}{V})^2$ term.

The van der Waals equation thus requires two coefficients a and b and these are taken as empirical parameters. If a and b are known for a gas, then the equation can be used just like the ideal gas law to calculate any one of {P, V, n and T} if the other three are known.

Dalton's Law of Partial Pressure More theory.

"The Total Pressure of a gas mixture was the sum of the Partial Pressure of each gas," i.e. $P_{total} = P_1 + P_2 + P_3 + \ldots\ldots P_n$

Partial pressure can be determined in two ways.
Using the ideal gas equation

> In this case, V, n, R, and T must be given, then calculate P by $PV = nRT$

Using mole fractions

> In this case, the total pressure and the moles or grams of each gas must be given, then $P_1 = X_1 (P_{total})$, where X_1 = mole fraction of the gas.

Dalton's law of partial pressures states that the total pressure exerted by the mixture of different gases in any gas volume will be, and is, equal to the sum of the partial pressures of each individual component in the overall gas mixture. Dalton's law also states that each individual component in any gas mixture exerts its own individual partial pressure, in the exact ratio as its mole fraction (or volume-based concentration) in that mixture. The relationship provides a way to determine the volume-based concentration of any individual gaseous component in a mixture of several other gases in air.

Practice Questions

Question 1

A given mass of a gas occupies 95cc under a pressure of 744 mm of mercury. What is the volume it will occupy at 760 mm pressure, if the temperature remains constant?

    A. 93 c.c

    B. 65 c.c

    C. 107 c.c

    D. 7 c.c

Question 2

A given mass of a gas occupies 240 ml at 27°C. What is the volume of the gas if its temperature is raised to 47°C?

    A. 540 ml

    B. 256 ml

    C. 300 ml

    D. 124 ml

Question 3

A gas cylinder containing cooking gas can withstand a pressure of 14.9 atmospheres. The pressure gauge of the cylinder indicates 12 atmospheres at 27°C. Due to a sudden fire in the building, its temperature starts rising. At what temperature will the cylinder explode?

    A. 99.5 °C

    B. 140 °C

    C. 30.5 °C

    D. 127 °C

Question 4

Hydrogen gas is collected in a glass tube over water as shown is the figure. The water level inside the tube is 40.8 mm higher than that outside. The barometric pressure is 730 mm Hg. The water vapour pressure at 29°C is found to be 30.0 mm Hg. What is the pressure of the dry hydrogen?

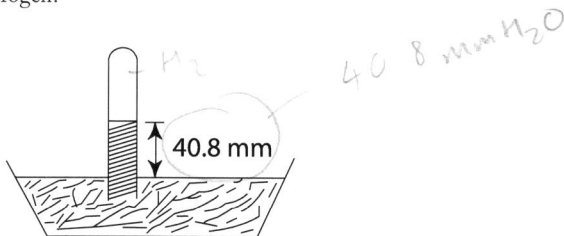

A. 659.2 mm Hg

B. 689.2 mm Hg

C. 697.0 mm Hg

D. 700.0 mm Hg

Question 5

A mixture of helium and argon contains 3 moles of He for every 2 moles of Ar. The partial pressure of argon is

    A. One third the total pressure

    B. Three-fifths the total pressure

    C. One half the total pressure

    D. Two-fifths the total pressure

Question 6

A mixture contains equal masses of methane and oxygen at the same temperature and pressure in an empty container. The ratio of partial pressure of methane to that of oxygen is

    A. 1:2

    B. 2:1

    C. 2:4

    D. 1:1

Question 7

A closed bulb contains inert He gas and solid NH_4Cl. All the NH_4Cl decomposes according to the following equation at 325°C

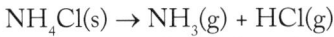

$$NH_4Cl(s) \rightarrow NH_3(g) + HCl(g)$$

At this temperature, the final total pressure in the bulb is 908 mm Hg. What is the partial pressure of $HCl(g)$ in the bulb at 325°C when the reaction is complete and partial pressure of He is 228 mm Hg?

    A. 340 mm Hg

    B. 680 mm Hg

    C. 568 mm Hg

    D. 760 mm Hg.

Question 8

When 2g of gaseous substance A is introduced into an initially evacuated flask at 25°C, the pressure is found to be 1.0 atm. The flask is evacuated and 3g of B is introduced, the pressure is found to be 0.5 atm at same temperature. The ratio, of M_A/M_B (molecular mass ratio of A to B) is

    A. 3:1

    B. 1:3

    C. 2:3

    D. 2:5

Question 9

Which one of the following is the units for the van der Waals constant 'a' ?

    A. L^2 atm mol^{-2}

    B. mol^2 L^{-2} atm

    C. L^2 mol^{-2} atm^{-1}

    D. atm^{-1}

Question 10

Which one of the following gas obeys the ideal gas law more closely than the other three gases?

    A. SO_2

    B. H_2

    C. CH_4

    D. CO_2

Question 11

Given the value of the van de Waals constant 'a' for the following gases:

Gas	'a' (L^2 mol^{-2} atm)
O_2	1.36
CO_2	3.59
C_2H_6	5.49
SO_2	6.72

Which one of the following gas has the strongest intermolecular forces of attraction?

    A. O_2

    B. CO_2

    C. C_2H_6

    D. SO_2

Question 12

For gas molecules

u_r = root mean square speed = $\sqrt{\dfrac{3k_bT}{m}}$

V_{mp} = most probable speed = $\sqrt{\dfrac{2k_bT}{m}}$

V_{av} = average speed = $\sqrt{\dfrac{8k_bT}{\pi m}}$

Which of the following is correct?

    A. $u_r > v_{mp} > v_{av}$

    B. $v_{mp} > v_{av} > u_r$

    C. $u_r > v_{av} > v_{mp}$

    D. $v_{av} > u_r > v_{mp}$

Question 13

At 298 K, the order of most probable speed of the following molecules $H_2(g)$, $N_2(g)$, $CH_4(g)$ and $O_2(g)$ is

    A. $N_2 > CH_4 > O_2 > H_2$

    B. $H_2 > CH_4 > N_2 > O_2$

    C. $H_2 > N_2 > O_2 > CH_4$

    D. $H_2 > N_2 > CH_4 > O_2$

Question 14

The number of collisions of Ar atoms with the walls of their container per unit time
  A. increases when the temperature decreases
  B. remains the same when CO_2 is added to the container at constant temperature.
  C. increases when CO_2 is added to the container at constant temperature.
  D. decreases when the average kinetic energy per molecule increases.

Question 15

At a given temperature, the ratio of root mean square speed: average speed: most probable speed is equal to
  A. 1.7:1.6:1:4
  B. 1.6:1.4:1.7
  C. 1.6:1.7:1:4
  D. 1:4:1.6:1.7

Question 16

According to Graham's law which states that the rate at which gases diffuse is inversely proportional to the square root of their densities. At a given temperature the ratio of

the rates of diffusion $\frac{r_A}{r_B}$ of gases A and B is given by which of the following?

A. $\left(\dfrac{M_A}{M_B}\right)^{\frac{1}{2}}$

B. $\left(\dfrac{M_A}{M_B}\right)$

C. $\left(\dfrac{M_B}{M_A}\right)^{\frac{1}{2}}$

D. $\left(\dfrac{M_B}{M_A}\right)$

Question 17

A bottle of dry NH_3 and a bottle of dry HCl connected through a long tube are opened simultaneously at both ends, the white NH_4Cl ring first formed will be

    A. at the centre of the tube

    B. near the hydrogen chloride bottle

    C. near the ammonia bottle

    D. throughout the length of the tube

Question 18

Given the van der Waals constant 'a' for the following gases

a :	0.211	1.39	3.59	4.17
Gas :	H_2	N_2	CO_2	NH_3

The most liquefiable gas is

    A. H_2

    B. N_2

    C. CO_2

    D. NH_3

Question 19

Which of the general shapes drawn below most closely represent the distribution of the velocities of molecules in a sample of gas?

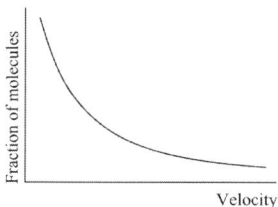

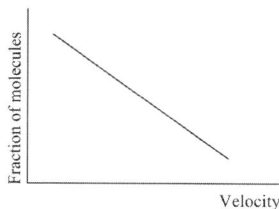

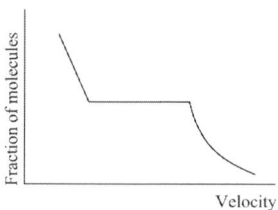

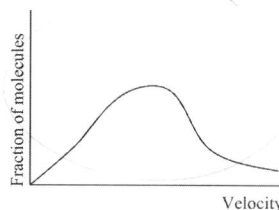

Question 20

Consider 1g of each of the following substances at S.T.P. which occupies the greatest volume?

(H = 1, F=19, S=32, O=16, Ne=20)

A. Fluorine 3 8

B. Hydrogen sulphide 3 3

C. Oxygen 3 2

D. Neon 2 0

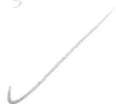

Solution

Question 1

Here,

P_1 = 744 mm P_2 = 760 mm

V_1 = 95 c.c. V_2 = ?

According to Boyle's Law, $P_1 \times V_1 = P_2 \times V_2$

$\therefore$ $744 \times 95 = 760 \times V_2$

$\therefore$ $V_2 = 744 \times \dfrac{95}{760} = 93 c.c$

Answer A.

Question 2

Here, V_1 = 240ml V_2 = ?

T_1 = 273 + 27 = 300

T_2 = 273 + 47 = 320

By Charles' Law,

$$\frac{V_1}{V_2} = \frac{T_1}{T_2}$$

Substituting the appropriate values, $\dfrac{240}{V_2} = \dfrac{300}{320}$

Or, $V_2 = 240 \times \dfrac{320}{300} = 256 ml$

Answer B.

Question 3

Since the gas is contained in a cylinder, its volume cannot increase with rise of temperature; instead the pressure will increase.

The gas cylinder will explode when the pressure of gas inside it rises to 14.9 atmospheres, the maximum it can withstand. Therefore,

P_1 = 12.0 atm. P_2 = 14.9 atm

T_1 = 273 + 27 = 300K T_2 = ?

Substituting these values in the above equation, $\dfrac{12}{300} = \dfrac{14.9}{T_2}$ or,

$T_2 = 14.9 \times \dfrac{300}{12} = 372.5K$

$\therefore$ The temperature in °C = 372.5 - 273

= 99.5°C

Answer A.

Question 4

Change the water height to the equivalent Hg height:
(Necessary conversion factor: 1 mm Hg = 13.6 mm H_2O)

$40.8 mmH_2O \times \dfrac{1mmHg}{13.6mmH_2O} = 3mmHg$

Adjust for the difference in height to get the gas pressure.
Pressure on the gas is 730 mm Hg – 3 mm Hg = 727 mm Hg.
Vapour pressure of H_2O at 29°C accounts for 30 mm Hg Pressure.
Therefore

727 mm Hg – 30 mm Hg = 697 mm Hg,

Answer C.

Question 5

The mole fraction of $Ar = \dfrac{2}{(2+3)} = \dfrac{2}{5}$

Partial pressure of $Ar = \dfrac{2}{5} \times P_{total}$

This is answer D.

Question 6

$$P = \frac{nRT}{V} \quad , \text{where} \quad n = \frac{g}{mw}$$

$$P_{CH_4} = \frac{gRT}{16V} \qquad (1)$$

$$P_{O_2} = \frac{gRT}{32V} \qquad (2)$$

Divide equation (1) by equation (2)

$$\frac{P_{CH_4}}{P_{O_2}} = \frac{32}{16} = 2:1$$

The answer is B.

Question 7

As number of moles of NH_3 = number of moles of HCl

Therefore $\quad P_{NH3} = P_{HCl}$

Total pressure = 908 = $P_{NH3} + P_{HCl} + P_{He}$ = 2 $P_{HCl} + P_{He}$

$$P_{HCl} = \frac{(908 - 228)}{2} = 340 mmHg$$

The answer is A.

Question 8

$$PV = \frac{w}{MRT}$$

$$1.0 \times V = \frac{2}{M_A RT} \qquad (1)$$

$$0.5 \times V = \frac{3}{M_B RT} \qquad (2)$$

Divide equation (2) by equation (1) gives

$$\frac{0.5}{1.0} = \frac{M_A}{M_B} \times \frac{3}{2}$$

$$\frac{M_A}{M_B} = \frac{2}{3} \times \frac{1}{2} = \frac{1}{3}$$

The answer is B.

Question 9

We known that $P = \dfrac{an^2}{V^2}$

$$a = \frac{PV^2}{n^2} = \frac{atmL^2}{mol^2}$$

L^2 atm mol^{-2}

The answer is A.

Question 10

The hydrogen gas behaves more ideally than the other three gases due to the absence of any intermolecular forces of attraction. The answer is B.

Question 11

The constant 'a' reflects the intermolecular attractions in real gases. The gas with the larger value of a will have larger forces of attraction. Looking at the values of 'a' for different gases gives answer D.

Question 12

The correct order is given in answer C. The most probable speed $v_{mp} = \sqrt{\dfrac{2k_bT}{m}}$; the average speed $v_{av} = \sqrt{\dfrac{8k_bT}{\pi m}}$; The root mean square speed $u_r = \sqrt{\dfrac{3k_bT}{m}}$ – since k_b, T, and m will be the same for all three equation, you simply need to compare

$$\sqrt{2} < \sqrt{\frac{8}{\pi}} < \sqrt{3}$$, which gives you the correct order.

Question 13

At a given temperature, most probable speed is inversely proportional to the square root of molar mass.
The molar mass of the given gases increases in the order

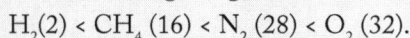

$H_2(2) < CH_4 (16) < N_2 (28) < O_2 (32)$.

Therefore, the correct order of their v_{mp} is

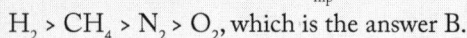

$H_2 > CH_4 > N_2 > O_2$, which is the answer B.

Question 14

The number of collision with the walls of the container increases with an increase in temperature so A is incorrect. At a given constant temperature, addition of any other gas does not change the number of collisions; this is the principle of Hess' Law. Therefore, the correct answer is B.

Question 15

$$\frac{u_r}{v_{av}} = \frac{\sqrt{\dfrac{3RT}{m}}}{\sqrt{\dfrac{8RT}{\pi m}}} = \sqrt{\frac{3\pi}{8}} = \frac{1.7}{1.6}$$

$$\frac{u_r}{v_{mp}} = \frac{\sqrt{\dfrac{3RT}{m}}}{\sqrt{\dfrac{2RT}{m}}} = \sqrt{\frac{3}{2}} = \frac{1.7}{1.4}$$

Hence

$$u_r : v_{av} : v_{mp} : 1.7 : 1.6 : 1.4$$

The answer is A.

Question 16

The question states that the rate of diffusion is inversely proportional to the square root of

the density. Therefore, $r = \dfrac{1}{\sqrt{density}}$

So for gases A and B, $\dfrac{r_A}{r_B} = \sqrt{\dfrac{d_B}{d_A}}$

Density is directly proportional to molar mass, therefore;

$$\frac{r_A}{r_B} = \sqrt{\frac{M_B}{M_A}}$$

The answer is C.

Question 17

The rate of diffusion of NH_3 is greater than the rate of diffusion of HCl since the molar mass of NH_3 is less than the molar mass of HCl. Therefore, the NH_3 will travel a longer distance in a tube than HCl and NH_4Cl will be formed near the HCl end.

The answer is B.

Question 18

A larger value of 'a' means a larger force of attraction between the gas molecules, so the gas with largest value of 'a' is the most compressible and most liquefiable because the attractive forces will hold it together. The answer is D. NH_3 is the most liquefiable gas out of these four given.

Question 19

The correct distribution curve should have few molecules with very low velocities, many molecules with velocities in an intermediate range and few molecules with really high velocities. This is represented by graph D.

Question 20

The substance of lowest relative molar mass will occupy the greatest volume. This is due to Avogadro's law which states that for gases under the same conditions, the molecular weight = 22.4 × vapour density. This means that the $d = \dfrac{mw}{22.4}$. Since $d = \dfrac{m}{V}$, and all of the gases have a mass of 1 g, $V = \dfrac{22.4}{mw}$. So, since the molecular weights of the compounds are $F_2(38)$, $H_2S(34)$, $O_2(32)$ and Ne(20), D is the correct answer.

GAMSAT Style Questions

Question 1-4

Boyle's Law states, "The volume of a given mass of a dry gas is inversely proportional to the pressure, if the temperature remains constant"

Graham's law of diffusion states, "The rate of diffusion of a gas is inversely proportional to the square root of its density"

Dalton's law states, "Total pressure exerted by a gaseous mixture is equal to the sum of the partial pressures of each individual component in a gas mixture"

1. Which of the following graph is NOT a correct representation of the Boyle's law?

A. B. C. D

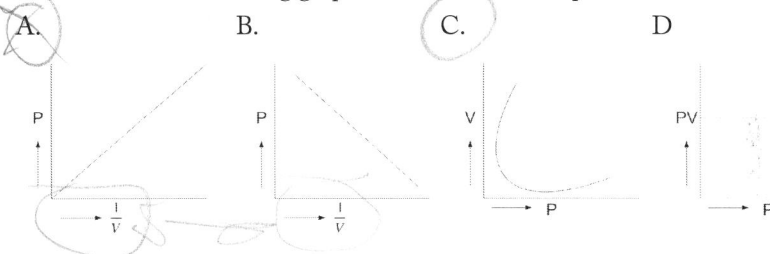

2. The density of gas X is four times that of gas Y. If the molecular weight of X is M, then the density of gas Y is

   A. $2M$

   B. $4M$

   C. $\dfrac{M}{2}$

   D. $\dfrac{M}{4}$

3. A closed vessel contains equal number of nitrogen and oxygen molecules at a pressure of P mm Hg. If nitrogen is removed from the system then the pressure will be (in mm Hg)

   A. P

   B. $2P$

   C. P^2

   D. $\dfrac{P}{2}$

4. When a gas is collected over water, to find the pressure of that gas, the pressure is corrected by

   A. Adding the vapour pressure of water

   B. Multiplying by the vapour pressure of water

   C. Subtracting the vapour pressure of water at that temperature

   D. Subtracting the temperature of the water from the vapour pressure

Question 5-8

Atmospheric pressure is defined as the force per unit area exerted against a surface by the weight of the air molecules above that surface. At sea level, it is 1 atm. When an object is taken underwater, for every 10 meters it goes underwater, there is 1 atm of pressure acting on it from the water in addition to the 1 atm of pressure from atmospheric pressure. Boyle's law states that there is an inverse relationship between pressure and volume. Thus if a gas filled container is taken underwater, the container will shrink. Similarly, when divers breath air from a scuba cylinder at depth, they will effectively have less air the deeper they descend. In this case, since the air is in an incompressible tank, the actual volume of the gas does not decrease, but since the air is being breathed at depth, and the lungs are compressible, the gas entering the lungs will be denser. Another important factor in diving involves Dalton's law of partial pressures that states that the sum of the partial pressure of each gas in a mixture will equal the total pressure. Certain gases such as oxygen can become toxic when breathed at depth, so the partial pressure of gases in scuba cylinders needs to be monitored.

5. A scuba tank is filled with 1400 L of compressed air at the surface. When the diver descends to 30 meters, what is the volume of air that will be available to the diver?

    A. 280L

    B. 350L

    C. 466.7L

    D. 700L

6. How may times more dense will a gas be if it is taken to a depth of 24 meters?

    A. 2.4 times

    B. 4.2 times

    C. 3.4 times

    D. 4.3 times

7. Decompression sickness or 'the bends" is a potentially fatal condition that results when excess nitrogen in the blood stream comes out of solution too quickly producing bubbles. When a diver breaths air at depth, the increase in the partial pressure of nitrogen causes excess nitrogen to dissolve in the blood stream. The blood becomes supersaturated with nitrogen. What circumstance would most likely result in a diver getting the bends?

    I. Driving up a mountain a few hours after diving

    II. Making a stop at 5 meters underwater for 3 minutes at the end of the dive

    III. Exceeding a depth of 40 meters

    IV. Ascending at a rate faster than the exhaled bubbles rise to the surface

    V. Remaining at a shallow depth for the duration of the dive

A. I, III, and V

B. II, III, and IV

C. I, III, and IV

D. All of the above

8. Nitrox is a special mixture of oxygen and nitrogen with oxygen percentages greater than that of air. It is used by divers to extend the amount of time they can spend at a particular depth by decreasing the chances of getting the bends. One problem encountered is that if oxygen is breathed at partial pressures above 1.4 atm, it can become toxic to the body. Consider a scuba tank filled with a 32% nitrox mixture. What is the maximum allowable depth for a diver using this mixture if they don't want to risk oxygen toxicity?

A. 34 meters

B. 21 meters

C. 57 meters

D. 44 meters

Solution

Question 1

STEP 1 = > What do you need to determine to solve the problem?

You need to determine which graph DOES NOT represent Boyle's law.

STEP 2 = > What relevant data provided in this problem is necessary in order to answer the question?

You are told that Boyle's Law states, "The volume of a given mass of a dry gas is inversely proportional to the pressure, if the temperature remains constant".

STEP 3 = > Use the relevant data to solve the question

According to Boyle's law $P = K \times \dfrac{1}{V}$

Therefore, the graph between P and $\dfrac{1}{V}$ at a given temperature is a straight line with positive slope, thus both Graph A and C can be correct. And at a given temperature, $PV = K$. Therefore PV vs. P graph will be the straight line parallel to the x-axis. Hence graph D can be correct too. The only incorrect graph of Boyle's law is B which shows that P and V are directly proportional.

Question 2

STEP 1 = > What do you need to determine to solve the problem?
You need to determine the molecular weight of gas Y.

STEP 2 = > What relevant data provided in this problem is necessary in order to answer the question?
You are told that the molecular weight of gas X is M and that density of gas X is 4 times that of gas Y. You are also told that Graham's law of diffusion states that the rate of diffusion of a gas is inversely proportional to the square root of its density.

STEP 3 = > Use the relevant data to solve the question
According to Graham's law of diffusion

$$\frac{r_1}{r_2} = \sqrt{\frac{d_2}{d_1}} \quad \text{and} \quad \frac{r_1}{r_2} = \sqrt{\frac{M_2}{M_1}}$$

the rate of diffusion is inversely proportional to both the square root of the density (d) and the square root of the molecular weight (M).

So, $\frac{M_2}{M_1} = \frac{d_2}{d_1}$

Let the density of gas Y be d_1, then the density of gas X will be $4d_1$,

$$\frac{4d_1}{d_1} = \frac{M}{M_Y}$$

$$4 = \frac{M}{M_Y}$$

$M_Y = \frac{M}{4}$, the answer is D.

Question 3

STEP 1 = > What do you need to determine to solve the problem?
You need to determine the pressure in a closed system containing oxygen and nitrogen once the nitrogen has been removed.

STEP 2 = > What relevant data provided in this problem is necessary in order to answer the question?
You know that the vessel originally contained equal amounts of nitrogen and oxygen, and that the original pressure of the system was *P*.

STEP 3 = > Use the relevant data to solve the question
Being a closed system, the volume V of the gas does not change. Using Dalton's Law
$P_{total} = P_1 + P_2 ...$ Since we are told that there are equal number of molecules of each gas,
$P_1 = P_2$
Given that the volume remains the same, the pressure would be P/2. The answer is D.

Question 4

STEP 1 = > What do you need to determine to solve the problem?
You need to determine the pressure the correction factor for finding the pressure of a gas when it is collected over water.

STEP 2 = > What relevant data provided in this problem is necessary in order to answer the question?
You are told that the gas is collected over water. You know that water possessed a certain vapour pressure at a specific temperature and pressure.

STEP 3 = > Use the relevant data to solve the question
The total pressure measured, P, is the sum of the partial pressure of the collected gas and the partial pressure of the gas phase of the liquid, which is its vapour pressure. If the liquid is water, as is most often the case, the pressure of the gas collected must be:
$$P_{(gas)} = P - P_{(H2O)}$$

Therefore the answer is C.

Question 5

STEP 1 = > What do you need to determine to solve the problem?
You need to determine the volume of air available at a depth of 30 meters.

STEP 2 = > What relevant data provided in this problem is necessary in order to answer the question?
You are told that Boyle's law states that there is an inverse relationship between pressure and volume. In addition, for every 10 meters underwater, the pressure increases by 1 atm.

STEP 3 = > Use the relevant data to solve the question
Use Boyle's law $P_1 \times V_1 = P_2 \times V_2$
The pressure at the surface is 1 atm
The pressure at 30 meters is 3 atm + 1 atm = 4 atm
The volume at the surface is 1400 L.
1 atm (1400 L) = 4 atm(x)
x = 350 L; the answer is B.

Question 6

STEP 1 = > What do you need to determine to solve the problem?
You need to determine the relationship between the density of a gas at the surface and at 24 meters below the surface.

STEP 2 = > What relevant data provided in this problem is necessary in order to answer the question?
You are given Boyle's law, and told that for every 10 meters underwater the pressure increases by 1 atm.

STEP 3 = > Use the relevant data to solve the question

Remember $d = \dfrac{m}{V}$

At 24 meters, the pressure is 3.4 atm, and therefore the volume is 3.4 times smaller than at the surface. The density is inversely proportional to the volume. Therefore, a 3.4x decrease in the volume will result in a 3.4x increase in the density. The answer is C.

Question 7

STEP 1 = > What do you need to determine to solve the problem?
You need to determine which circumstances are likely to result in the bends.

STEP 2 = > What relevant data provided in this problem is necessary in order to answer the question?
You are given that the bends is caused when the nitrogen that dissolves in the blood stream at depth comes out of solution too quickly.

STEP 3 = > Use the relevant data to solve the question
When the concentration of a gas above a liquid is less than the concentration of the gas in the liquid, the gas will come out of solution. If the difference is too great, the liquid is said to be supersaturated and bubbles of the gas will form as it comes out of solution. Because at depth the partial pressure of nitrogen is greater than at the surface, as a diver ascends, the amount of nitrogen outside of the blood will decrease, and nitrogen will begin to come out of solution. If this is done slowly enough, then the risk of developing the bends is minimal. In addition, if a diver sits at a depth shallower than the maximum depth for a period of time, it allows the nitrogen in the system more time to equilibrate thereby decreasing the risk of developing the bends. So, lets examine the statements

    I. Ascending to altitude on land has the same effect as ascending from depth. The rapid decrease in atmospheric pressure associated with going up to a higher altitude could cause nitrogen supersaturation – True.

    II. Making a stop at 5 meters for 3 minutes allows the body a bit of time to equilibrate the nitrogen in the blood stream with that at the lower partial pressure than the previous depth experience – False.

    III. The deeper you go, the more nitrogen that will deposit in your system, at this depth the partial pressure of nitrogen is 5 times that at the surface – True.

    IV. Ascending too quickly does not allow the body time to equilibrate the nitrogen outside the blood with that dissolved in the blood – True.

    V. Staying shallow means that the partial pressure difference is small, therefore, it will take less time to equilibrate.

The correct answer is C.

Question 8

STEP 1 = > What do you need to determine to solve the problem?
You need to determine the maximum allowable depth for a diver using a 32% oxygen
containing nitrox mixture.

STEP 2 = > What relevant data provided in this problem is necessary in order to answer
the question?
You are told that oxygen partial pressures above 1.4 can be toxic. In addition, you are given
that the mixture contains 32% oxygen.

STEP 3 = > Use the relevant data to solve the question
The partial pressure of oxygen = fraction of oxygen * the total pressure.
Therefore, if 1.4 bar is the highest P_{O2} that can be obtained, $1.4 = 0.32 P_{total}$
P_{total} = 4.4 atm.
For every 10 meters, the pressure increases by 1 atm. So, 4.4 atm – 1 atm = 3.4 atm – which
is the pressure exerted by the water only. This corresponds to a depth of 34 meters.
The answer is A.

Chapter 5: **Solutions**

Key Concept: Solution

A solution is a homogeneous mixture of two or more kinds of molecular or ionic species, or a combination of both. Solutions may be composed of any combination of the three states of matter- gases, liquids and solids; but they always consist of a single phase. In a solution, all of the particles exist as individual molecules or ions. Solutions do not settle out if left to sit undisturbed. In addition, there are special types of solutions termed colloid, sol, and gel where the particle size is much larger than the individual molecules, however the particle size is so small that the mixture never settles out.

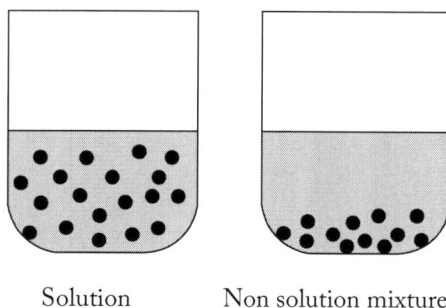

Solution   Non solution mixture

The components of a solution are called the solvent and the solute. The component present in greater amount is called the solvent, and the other component(s) the solute(s). It may be noted that the solvent has the same physical state as the solution itself. In the case where the substances are in equal amounts, water or the liquid substance is the solvent. Concentration refers to how much solute is dissolved in the solution. A dilute solution is one which has little solute, and a concentrated solution has a lot of dissolved solute. These are qualitative terms, while molarity and molality which will be discussed later are quantitative ways of describing concentration.

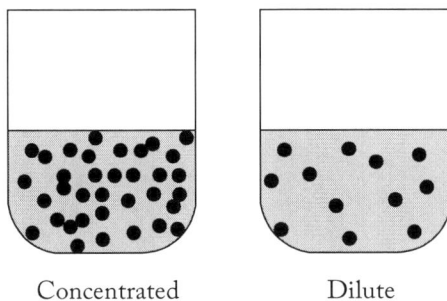

Concentrated   Dilute

Key Concept: Miscibility and Solubility

Miscibility is the ability of two substances to mix together. It is important to remember that "like dissolves like." Both water and ethanol are polar molecules with hydrogen bonding between molecules abilities. The similarity of the two molecules results in solutions where the water molecules and CH_3CH_2OH are interchangeable. Likewise, Organic compounds like n-hexane, C_6H_{14}, and dodecane, $C_{12}H_{26}$, are miscible in one another. The non-polar molecules are attracted to one another through London forces (dispersion forces).

Any substance that can form a 0.1 M solution or greater is referred to as soluble, while any substance that fails to reach 0.1 M is insoluble. This value was chosen because VERY FEW substances have their maximum solubility near 0.1 M and almost every substance of importance in chemistry is either more or less soluble. When it comes to solubility in water, certain rules apply.

- All alkali metals and ammonium compounds are soluble
- All acetate, perchlorate, and nitrate compounds are soluble
- Silver, lead, and mercury compounds are insoluble
- Chlorides, bromides, and iodides are soluble
- Carbonates, hydroxides, oxides, phosphates, silicates, and sulfides are insoluble
- Sulfates are soluble except calcium and barium

These rules apply in order, so $PbSO_4$ is insoluble since rule 3 comes before rule 6. As always, there are a few exceptions to these rules, but they are very rare.

Concentrations

Concentrations of solutions, common terms used to describe the concentrations (or strengths) of solutions are:

      (1) Mole fraction

      (2) Molarity

      (3) Molality

      (4) Normality

Key Concept: Mole Fraction

Mole fraction is the ratio of the number of moles of a particular component of the solution to the total number of moles of all components. If N_a represents the number of moles of the solute and N_b the number of moles of solvent in a two-component solution, then the mole fraction of the solute is

$$Xa = \frac{Na}{(Na + Nb)}$$

and the mole fraction of the solvent is

$$Xb = \frac{Nb}{(Na + Nb)}$$

Obviously, Xa + Xb = 1. Mole fraction has no units.

Key Concept: Molarity

The molarity, M, of solution is the number of moles of solute per litre of solution. For example, a 2M solution of NaCl would have 2×58.5g/mol of NaCl in a sufficient amount of water to produce 1L of solution. To calculate the M of a solution, you need to know the weight of the solute plus the molecular weight (m.wt.) of the solute, and the total volume. For example, the M of a solution of when 100g of NaCl is dissolved in 5L of water would be:

      [Weight of solute/ m.wt. of solute]/Volume =M (mol/L)

$$\frac{\frac{100g}{58.5g/mol}}{5L} = 0.34M$$

Key Concept: Molality

The molality, m, of a solution is the number of moles of solute per 1000g (or 1 kg) of solvent. For example, 1 mole of NaCl (i.e. 58.5g of NaCl) dissolved in 1000g of water gives a 1 molal aqueous solution of a sodium chloride.

Suppose you have 1.00 mole of sucrose (mw~342.3g/mol) and mix it with 1 L of water. You keep adding water, dissolving and stirring until the entire solid is gone. What would be the molality of this solution? Note: 1L of water weighs 1000g (density of water = 1g/ml).

$$\text{So,} \quad Molality = \frac{1.00mol}{1.00kg} = 1mol/kg = 1m$$

Key Concept: Normality

When you need to compare solutions on the basis of concentration of specific ions or the amount of charge that the ions have, a different measure of concentration can be very useful. It is called normality. The normality of a solution is simply a multiple of the molarity of the solution. Generally, the normality of a solution is just one, two or three times the molarity. In rare cases it can be four, five, six or even seven times as much.

Quantitatively, the normality of a solution N, is the number of gram equivalents of a solute in one litre of solution.

That is, Normality, N = gram equivalents (E) / Litres of solution (V)

For an acid solution, n is the number of H^+ provided by a formula unit of acid. For example: A 3 M H_2SO_4 solution is the same as a 6 N H_2SO_4 solution.

For a basic solution, n is the number of OH^- provided by a formula unit of base. For example: A 1 M $Ca(OH)_2$ solution is the same as a 2N $Ca(OH)_2$ solution.

Key Concept: Relationship between Normality and Molarity

Normality and molarity are interchangeable according to the following relationship:

$$Nomality = Molarity \times \frac{mw}{Eq.wt.}$$

$$Molarity = Normality \times \frac{Eq.wt.}{mw}$$

Remember, N is never less than M

Key Concept: Raoult's Law

All liquids (and, volatile solids) give off vapour consisting of molecules of the substance. If the substance is in an enclosed space, the pressure of the vapour will reach a maximum, which depends only upon the nature of the substance and the temperature. This maximum pressure is called the vapour pressure of the substance at the given temperature.

"For a solution of volatile liquids, the partial vapour pressure of each component in the solution is directly proportional to its mole fraction". This statement in referred to as Raoult's law. It does not apply if the mixture of volatile liquids does not form a solution.

Consider an ideal solution of two liquids A and B. Let their mole fractions be X_A and X_B respectively. Then their partial pressures P_A and P_B respectively above the solution will be proportional to their respective mole fractions in solution. That is,

$$P_A \propto X_A \text{ and } P_B \propto X_B$$

Result show that the relationship between the partial pressures and the mole fractions can be written as:

$$P_A = P^o_A X_A \text{ and } P_B = P^o_B X_B$$

Where P^o_A is the vapour pressure of pure A and P^o_B is the vapour pressure of pure B. So, the proportionality constant is the vapour pressure of the pure component.

Therefore, at a given temperature, the vapour pressure of a component in a solution is equal to the product of its mole fraction and the vapour pressure of the pure component. A solution, which obeys Raoult's law, occurs when the vapour pressures (total and partial) of the solution and its components are lower than those for ideal solution. Such solutions are formed with the evolution of heat.

Positive deviation from Raoult's law occurs when the vapour pressures (total and partial) of the solution and its components are higher than those for ideal solution. Such solutions are formed with the absorption of heat.

-->*Quick Facts:* Properties of Solutions

The colligative properties of solutions are dependent only on the number of particles of solute and not the type of particle or the mass of material in solution. They are as follows:
- The solution shows an increase in osmotic pressure between it and a reference solution as the amount of solute is increased.
- The solution shows an increase in boiling point as the amount of solute is increased.
- The solution shows a decrease in melting point as the amount of solute is increased.
- A solution of a solid non-volatile solute in a liquid solvent shows a decrease in vapour pressure above the solution as the amount of solute is increased.

NOTE: KNOW THESE PROPERTIES!!!

GAMSAT Style Questions

Question 1
Sodium hydroxide and hydrochloric acid combine to make sodium chloride (table salt) and water. 14 mL of 0.1 M sodium hydroxide is added to an excess of acid.

m.wt Na = 23g/mol
m.wt O = 16g/mol
m.wt. Cl = 35.5g/mol
m.wt. H = 1g/mol

How many grams of table salt are created?
A. 1.4×10^{-3}g
B. 0.08g
C. 0.014g
D. 2.4×10^{-5}g

Question 2

Consider four different solutions consisting of the same solute and solvent.

Solution	b.p
A	105.7 °C
B	92.5 °C
C	137.3 °C
D	116.8 °C

Given the above data, what can you determine about the relative concentrations of the four different solutions?

      A. B > A > D > C

      B. C > D > A > B

      C. C > A > B > D

      D. There is not enough information to determine the relative amount of solute in the different solutions

Solution

Question 1

STEP 1 = > What do you need to determine to solve the problem?
The number of grams of table salt created by the reaction of sodium hydroxide with hydrochloric acid.

STEP 2 = > What relevant data provided in this problem is necessary in order to answer the question?
You know that you have 14 mL of a 0.1M solution of NaOH and it is reacted with an excess of HCl. It tells you that this reaction produces sodium chloride (table salt) and water. You are also provided with the molecular weights of all elements involved in the reaction allowing you to calculate the m.wt. for any molecule in the reaction.

STEP 3 = > Use the relevant data to solve the question
First, you need to write out and balance the reaction as shown:
$NaOH + HCl \rightarrow NaCl + H_2O$

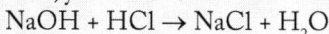

Next you know that the NaOH is the limiting reagent since the reaction is carried out in an excess of HCl, so now you need to figure out how many moles of NaOH you have. You should recall that M = mol/L .

0.1M NaOH * 0.014L (convert from mL to L) = 1.4×10^{-3} mol of NaOH. Since the ratio of NaOH consumed to NaCl formed is 1:1, this means that 1.4×10^{-3} mol of NaCl are formed. Now you simply need to convert mol of NaCl to g of NaCl using the m.wt.
1.4×10^{-3} mol NaCl × 58.5 g/mol (35.5g + 23 g) = 0.08 g. The correct answer is B.

Question 2

STEP 1 = > What do you need to determine to solve the problem
You need to determine the relative concentrations of the four different solutions.

STEP 2 = > What relevant data provided in this problem is necessary in order to answer the question?
The question provides you with a table containing the four different solutions and their boiling points.

STEP 3 = > Use the relevant data to solve the question
To answer this question, you need to recall one of the four colligative properties. As the amount of solute increases, the boiling point increases. Therefore, the more concentrated the solution is, the higher its boiling point will be. Hence you simply now need to order the solutions from highest to lowest boiling point. The answer is B.

Chapter 6: **Vapour Pressure**

Key Concepts: Vapour Pressure

The **vapour pressure** of a compound is defined as the pressure at any given temperature (standard T is 25 °C) of a vapour (gas) in equilibrium with its liquid. When the liquid is pure, the resulting pressure is called the saturation vapour pressure and given the symbol $P_l^{'}$, where subscript '1' reminds us that the vapour is in equilibrium with the liquid (or sub-cooled liquid phase, see below) of the solute.

If the compound is a crystalline solid at the temperature of interest, then the saturation vapour pressure is notated by P_s^{o}.

Pre solid compounds can either vapourize (volatilize) directly, which is called sublimation, or they can first melt to the liquid phase and then volatilize. In either case, the energy required is the same.

To give you a better idea of vapour pressure, here is a step-by-step explanation that will help. First, imagine a closed box that is several litres in size. It has rigid walls and is totally empty of all substances. Now, liquid is injected into the box, but does not fill it. So, what happens to the liquid? Some, or maybe even all of the liquid will evaporate into a gas filling the empty space. Supposing that only some of the liquid evaporates, the gas present above the liquid is called its vapour, and this vapour creates a pressure called the vapour pressure. The key here is that the gas must be in contact with the liquid (or solid) at all times.

So, you may be wondering how the molecules of the liquid (or solid) become molecules of gas. Each molecule in the liquid has its own particular energy. The energy is distributed according to the Maxwell-Boltzmann distribution. Now, it's not really important to know what that is, but the important point here is that some of the molecules have a large amount of energy compared to the average. If one of these high energy molecules happens to be sitting at the surface of the liquid, it is of particular interest. Because to their energy, the molecules are all in motion, but none of them have enough energy to break free from the attractive force they have for each other. Now, if the high energy surface molecule moves up and away from the surface and happens to have enough energy to break the attractive forces, it could become a molecule of gas and a vapour and resulting vapour pressure is formed. As this happens to more molecules, the vapour pressure increases. At some point however, the vapour pressure will stop increasing and remain at a fixed value. Now what is happening is that as more and more molecules leave the surface, some start to return. When the number leaving and returning is equal, the pressure stays constant and the system is in equilibrium.

Two important things to note regarding vapour pressure
- Vapour pressure depends ONLY on temperature
- Increasing the amount of liquid WILL NOT increase the vapour pressure

Key Concepts: Phase diagrams

Figure 1a shows a phase diagram for water and Figure 1b illustrates typical vapour pressure characteristics of a substance.

PHASE DIAGRAM
Figure 1a shows a phase diagram for water and Figure 1b illustrates typical vapour pressure characteristics of a substance

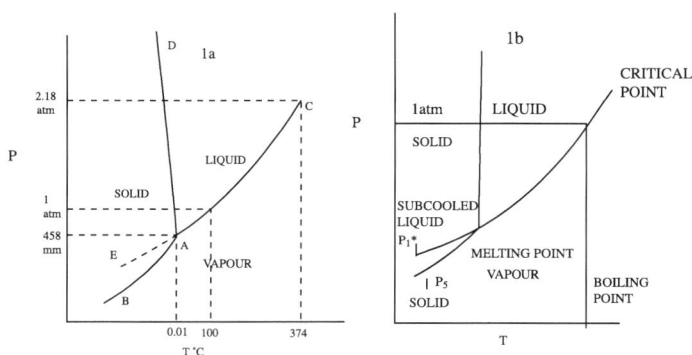

Curve AC	Vapour pressure curve of liquid water. At any given T there is only one pressure (P_1) at which water vapour is in equilibrium with liquid water. The curve separates the liquid region from the vapour region.
Point C	Critical point beyond which only the vapour phase exists.
Curve AB	Sublimation pressure curve (P_s) of the solid (ice).
Curve AD	Liquid-solid equilibrium. {Note that the freezing T decreases with increasing P for water. For most compounds increasing P has no effect on freezing point, or causes an increase in T.}
Point A	The Triple point where water vapour, liquid water, and solid ice are in equilibrium. {For some compounds this point also corresponds to the melting point, which is measured at 1 atm, but not for water.}
Curve AE	This is the vapour pressure curve for sub-cooled water (P_1°), which is an extension of curve AC, and is dotted because the system is meta-stable. NOTE: The sub-cooled-liquid vapour pressure P_1° is greater than P_s°.

Practice Questions

In order to have a better understanding on the principles, try to solve these questions.

Question 1–16

1. The mole fraction of H_2SO_4 (MW = 98) in a 98% by mass H_2SO_4 solution is (MW of H_2O =18)

   A. 1.0

   B. 0.9

   C. 0.11

   D. 0.010

2. The mole fraction of water in a mixture consisting of 9.0g water and 120g acetic acid, CH_3COOH is

   A. 0.8

   B. 0.2

   C. 1.0

   D. 0.5

3. The mole fraction of water in a 20% aqueous solution of H_2O_2 is

   A. $\frac{68}{77}$

   B. $\frac{77}{68}$

   C. $\frac{9}{68}$

   D. $\frac{9}{77}$

4. What is the mole fraction of H_2 in a gaseous mixture containing 1.0g H_2, and 8.0g of oxygen?

   A. $\frac{50}{75}$

   B. $\frac{75}{50}$

   C. $\frac{5.0}{90}$

   D. $\frac{1.0}{9.0}$

5. In an equimolar mixture of methanol, CH_3OH (MW = 32) and ethanol, C_2H_5OH (MW = 46), the mass of ethanol is
    A. 46.0g
    B. 23.0g
    C. 92.0g
    D. 4.6g

6. An aqueous solution of acetone, CH_3COCH_3, is 10.00% acetone by weight the mole percentage of acetone in this solution is
    A. 3.332%
    B. 5.000%
    C. 10.00%
    D. 11.11%

7. In a solution of 7.8g of benzene (C_6H_6) and 46 g of methyl benzene ($C_6H_5CH_3$), the mole fraction of benzene is

    A. $\dfrac{1}{6}$

    B. $\dfrac{1}{5}$

    C. $\dfrac{1}{3}$

    D. $\dfrac{1}{2}$

8. A solution is prepared by dissolving 12.2g of solid benzoic acid, C_6H_5COOH, in 97.5 mL of benzene of density 0.80g mL^{-1}. The mole fraction of benzoic acid in this solution is
    A. $\dfrac{10}{11}$

    B. $\dfrac{1}{2}$

    C. $\dfrac{3}{4}$

    D. $\dfrac{1}{11}$

9. The molarity of a 500cm³ solution containing 4g of NaOH (m.wt. H = 1, O = 16, Na = 23) is

    A. 0.1

    B. 0.2

    C. 3.0

    D. 0.50

10. 200cm³ solution of sodium sulfate, Na_2SO_4, contains 3.01×10^{23} Na^+ ions. The molarity of the solution is

    A. 1.25

    B. 2.5

    C. 3.0

    D. 0.50

11. The molarity of a solution of Na_2CO_3, containing 10.6 g of Na_2CO_3, in a half litre solution is

    A. 0.20 M

    B. 0.020 M

    C. 2.0 M

    D. 20 M

12. If 49 grams of H_2SO_4 is mixed with enough water to make 500 mL of solution, then the molarity of the solution is

    A. 0.25

    B. 0.50

    C. 0.75

    D. 1.0

13. A 5 M solution of HCl would have how many moles of H^+ ion in 0.1 L?

    A. 5.0

    B. 2.5

    C. 1.0

    D. 0.5

14. How many grams of NaCl will be needed to make 100 cm³ of 2 M solution? (atomic masses : (Na = 23, Cl = 35.5)

    A. 5.85

    B. 11.7

    C. 58.5

    D. 117

15. How many grams of NaOH are needed to make 100 cm³ of a 5% solution?

    A. 2

    B. 5

    C. 20

    D. 95

16. 50 mL of 0.1 M HCl and 50 mL of 0.050 M H_2SO_4 is mixed. What is the molarity of the final solution?

    A. 0.025

    B. 0.250

    C. 0.075

    D. There is no single value of molarity

Solutions

Question 1-16

1. 100 g of solution contains 98 g H_2SO_4.

   Therefore, number of moles of H_2SO_4, $n_B = \dfrac{98g}{98g/mol} = 1mol$

   And the number of moles of water, $n_A = \dfrac{2g}{18g/mol} = 0.11mol$

   The mole fraction of $H_2SO_4 = \dfrac{1}{(1+0.11)} = 0.9$. The answer is B.

2. nWater $= \dfrac{9.0}{18} = 0.5$

   nCH₃COOH$= \dfrac{120}{60} = 2.0$

   ∴ mole fraction of water is $\dfrac{0.5}{(2.0+0.5)}$ = 0.2, which is answer B.

3. $nH_2O_2 = \dfrac{20}{34} = 0.59$; $nH_2O \dfrac{80}{18} = 4.44$

    Mole fraction of $H_2O = \dfrac{4.44}{(4.44+0.59)}$ = 0.88

    Therefore the answer is A.

4. Mole fraction of $H_2 = \dfrac{\dfrac{1.0}{2}}{(\dfrac{1.0}{2}+\dfrac{8.0}{32})} = \dfrac{32}{48} = \dfrac{2}{3} = \dfrac{50}{75}$

   The answer is A.

5. The mole fraction of ethanol is 0.5. It is an equimolar mixture, containing 1 mole of ethanol. Therefore, the mass of ethanol is 1 mole × 46 g mol⁻¹ = 46.0.g. The answer is A.

6. $nAcetone = \dfrac{10}{58}$; $nH_2O = \dfrac{90}{18}$;

$$x\,Acetone = \dfrac{\dfrac{10}{58}}{(\dfrac{10}{58} + \dfrac{90}{18})} = 0.0338$$

Mole percentage of acetone = 0.338 X 100 = 3.38 % which is very close to answer A.

7. n Benzene = $\dfrac{7.8}{78}$ = 0.1; n Methylbenzene = $\dfrac{46}{92}$ = 0.5

$\dfrac{0.1}{(0.1 + 0.5)} = \dfrac{1}{6}$. The answer is A.

8. Molecular weight of benzene = 78g

n Benzoic acid = $\dfrac{12.2}{122} = 0.1$

n Benzene = $97.5 \times \dfrac{0.80}{78} = 1.0$

x Benzoic acid = $\dfrac{0.1}{(0.1 + 1.0)} = \dfrac{0.1}{1.1} = \dfrac{1}{11}$. The answer is D.

9. $M = \dfrac{n}{V} = \dfrac{\dfrac{4}{40mol}}{0.5L} = 0.2$. The answer B.

10. $2 \times 6.02 \times 10^{23}$ Na^+ ions are contained in 1 mole Na_2SO_4

$\therefore 3.01 \times 10^{23}$ Na^+ ion will be contained in $\dfrac{3.01 \times 10^{23}}{(2 \times 6.02 \times 10^{23})} = \dfrac{1}{4}$ mol Na_2SO_4

V= 200 cm³ = 200 mL = 0.200 L. Therefore, Molarity of the solution is

$M = \dfrac{\dfrac{1}{4}}{0.2} = 1.25$, answer A.

11. V= 0.5 L

$$n\ Na_2CO_3 = \frac{10.6g}{106g/mol} = 0.1\ mol$$

$$M = \frac{n}{V} = \frac{0.1mol}{0.5L} = 0.20M$$, answer A.

12. Number of moles of H_2SO_4 = $\frac{49g}{98g/mol} = \frac{1}{2}mol$

Volume of solution is 500 mL or 0.500 L. Therefore, the molarity of the solution is .05/0.5=1.0. The answer is D.

13. $M = \frac{n}{V}$

The number of moles of H^+ = number of mole of HCl

= $M_{HCl} \times V_{HCl}$

= 5 × 0.1 = 0.5, which is answer D.

14. Number of moles of NaCl needed to make 100 cm^3 solution of strength 2 M is

2M = 2 mol/L, so to make 0.1 L a 2M NaCl solution, you would need

2 × 0.1 =0.2 mole of NaCl.

MW NaCl = 23 + 35.5 = 58.5 g/mol

Mass of NaCl needed for a 2M solution will be

= 0.2 mol × 58.5g/mol = 11.7, the answer is B.

15. One litre of water is 1000 grams

a 5% solution of NaOH means there are 50 grams of NaOH in a one litre of solution.

100 grams of solution means that there is $\frac{1}{10}$ th of 1 litre. (1 litre divided by 10)

Therefore to obtain the number of grams of NaOH in 100 grams of solution.

we must multiply the amount of NaOH in 1 liter by $\frac{1}{10}$.

$$50 \times \frac{1}{10} = 5$$

5.0 g of Na OH are required which is answer B.

16. Since HCl and H_2SO_4 are both strong acids they do not react with each other.

In solution containing more than one solute, molarity of the solution is the number of moles of solute per litre of the solution.

In the solution of HCl and H_2SO_4 there are H^+ ions, SO_4^{2-} and Cl^- ions in the solution. So molarity of the solution is the concentration of each ion in the solution.

Therefore, there is no single value of molarity.

The answer is D.

GAMSAT Style Questions

Questions 1–4

A solution is a homogeneous dispersion of two or more kinds of molecular or ionic species, or a combination of both. Solutions may be composed of any combination of the three states of matter-gases, liquids and solids- but they always consist of a single phase.

Molarity. The molarity, M, of solution is the number of moles of solute per litre of solution.

Molality. The molality, m, of a solution is the number of moles of solute per 1000g of solvent.

1. A 0.01 M solution of $KMnO_4$ reacts with acidified ferrous sulfate solution according to the equation
   $$MnO_4^- + 5Fe^{2+} + 8H^+ \rightarrow Mn^{2+} + 5\ Fe^{3+} + 4H_2O$$
   The normality of the $KMnO_4$ solution originally was
   A. 2 N
   B. $\dfrac{1}{100}$ N
   C. $\dfrac{1}{2}$ N
   D. $\dfrac{1}{20}$ N

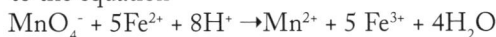

2. 1L solution contains 4.0 g of NaOH in it. The difference between molarity and the normality is

    A. 0.10

    B. zero

    C. 0.05

    D. 0.20

3. Addition of a solute to a given solvent in a closed container

    A. decreases the rate of condensation

    B. decreases the rate of evaporation

    C. increases the rate of evaporation

    D. decreases both the rate of evaporation and condensation

4. The normal boiling point of the solution is the temperature at which the vapour pressure of the solution is

    A. equal to the external solution

    B. equal to 76 mm Hg

    C. equal to 2.0 atmosphere

    D. equal to one atmosphere

Question 5 - 8

Use the following additional information for the following questions.

"For a solution of volatile liquids, the partial vapour pressure of each component in the solution is directly proportional to its mole fraction". This is referred to as Raoult's law. Consider an ideal solution of two liquids A and B. Let their mole fractions be X_A and X_B respectively. Then their partial pressures P_A and P_B respectively above the solution will be proportional to their respective mole fractions in solution. That is,

$$P_A \propto X_A \text{ and } P_B \propto X_B$$

Result showed that these relationships could be put as

$$P_A = P^o_A X_A \text{ and } P_B = P^o_B X_B$$

Where P^o_A is the vapour of pure A and P^o_B the vapour pressure of pure B. That is, the proportionality constant is the vapour pressure of pure component.

5. At 293 K, the vapour pressure of pure benzene is 75 mm Hg and that of pure toluene is 22 mmHg. The vapour pressure of the solution which contains 20.0 mol% benzene and 80.0 mol % toluene is

    A. 32.6 mmHg

    B. 64.4 mmHg

    C. 97.0 mmHg

    D. 3.26mmHg

6. A liquid is in equilibrium with its vapour at its boiling point. On average, the molecules in the two phases have equal

    A. potential Energy

    B. inter-molecular forces

    C. kinetic Energy

    D. total energy

7. The vapour pressure of a liquid in a closed container depends upon

    A. the amount of liquid

    B. surface area of the container

    C. temperature

    D. none of these

8. At high altitudes, water boils at a temperature less than 100°C because

    A. atmospheric pressure is low

    B. temperature is low

    C. atmospheric pressure is high

    D. temperature is high

Questions 9-10

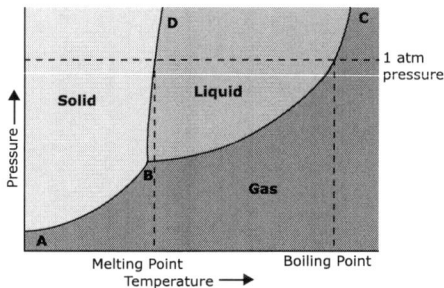

Melting Point   Boiling Point
Temperature ⟶

Examine the above phase diagram

9. What information CANNOT be obtained from the following diagram?

     A. The vapour pressure of a substance at a given temperature

     B. The sublimation point of a substance at a give temperature

     C. The temperature and pressure beyond which the substance exists only in the vapour phase

     D. The types of intermolecular forces present at a given temperature

10. Raoult's law states that given an ideal solution of two liquids A and B. Let their mole fractions be X_A and X_B respectively. Then their partial pressures P_A and P_B respectively above the solution will be proportional to their respective mole fractions in solution. That is,

$$P_A \propto X_A \text{ and } P_B \propto X_B$$

Result showed that these relationships could be put as

$$P_A = P^o_A X_A \text{ and } P_B = P^o_B X_B$$

Where P^oA is the vapour of pure A and P^oB the vapour pressure of pure B. That is, the proportionality constant is the vapour pressure of pure component.
The vapour pressure above a glucose-water solution at 25°C is 23.8 torr. The vapour pressure of water at 25°C is 30.5 torr. What is the mole fraction of glucose in the solution?

     A. 0.77

     B. 0.22

     C. 0.44

     D. 0.55

Solution

Question 1
STEP 1 = > What do you need to determine to solve the problem?
You need to determine the normality of the original $KMnO_4$ solution.

STEP 2 = > What relevant data provided in this problem is necessary in order to answer the question?
You are given the chemical equation for the reaction of $KMnO_4$ with acidified ferrous sulfate solution. In addition, you are given the definition of Molarity – it is the number of moles per litre of solution.

STEP 3 = > Use the relevant data to solve the question
You need to recall the relationship between Molarity and Normality. Normality (N) = Molarity × no. of electrons gained or lost. So you need to determine the number of electrons gained or lost for the reaction. In the case of this reaction, there is a 5 electrons difference because of the change of Fe from +2 to +3; (so since there are 5 of each, it would be a change from +2(5) = 10 to +3(5) = 15). Therefore, N = .01 × 5 = $\frac{1}{20}$ which is answer D.

Question 2
STEP 1 = > What do you need to determine to solve the problem?
You need to determine the difference between the molarity and normality of the NaOH solution.

STEP 2 = > What relevant data provided in this problem is necessary in order to answer the question?
You are told that you have a 1L solution containing 4g of NaOH.

STEP 3 = > Use the relevant data to solve the question
There is only one replaceable OH^- in NaOH. Therefore, the normality and molarity will be the same and their difference will be zero. The answer is B.

Question 3
STEP 1 = > What do you need to determine to solve the problem?
You need to determine the effect of adding solute to a solution in a closed container.

STEP 2 = > What relevant data provided in this problem is necessary in order to answer the question?
This question relied on you to recall certain useful facts presented earlier in this section.

STEP 3 = > Use the relevant data to solve the question
Addition of solute decreases the number of solvent molecules going into the vapour state and decreases the rate of evaporation. The answer is B.

Question 4

STEP 1 = > What do you need to determine to solve the problem?
You need to determine what is true about the vapour pressure at the boiling point of a solution.

STEP 2 = > What relevant data provided in this problem is necessary in order to answer the question?
Again, you need to rely on prior knowledge of chemistry to answer this question. Remember they are asking about the NORMAL boiling point.

STEP 3 = > Use the relevant data to solve the question
A boiling point is the temperature at which the vapour pressure is equal to the external pressure. When external pressure is equal to one atmosphere, then the temperature is known as the normal boiling point. The correct answer is D.

Question 5

STEP 1 = > What do you need to determine to solve the problem?
You need to determine the vapour pressure of a solution that contains 20.0 mol % benzene and 80.0 mol % toluene.

STEP 2 = > What relevant data provided in this problem is necessary in order to answer the question?
You are told that the vapour pressure of each component in a solution will be equal to the mole fraction × the pressure of the pure substance. The total vapour pressure will be the sum of its components.

STEP 3 = > Use the relevant data to solve the question
According to Raoult's Law

$$P = P^{\circ}_B X_B + P^{\circ}_T X_T$$
$$= 75 \times 0.20 + 22 \times 0.08 = 32.6 \text{ mm Hg}$$

The answer is A.

Question 6

STEP 1 = > What do you need to determine to solve the problem?
You need to determine what is true about the molecules of a solution that is at equilibrium with its liquid and vapour phase (at the boiling point).

STEP 2 = > What relevant data provided in this problem is necessary in order to answer the question?
You need to recall the definitions of kinetic energy, potential energy, total energy, and intermolecular forces.

STEP 3 = > Use the relevant data to solve the question
When a liquid is in equilibrium with its vapours at its boiling point, on an average, the

molecules in these two phases will have equal kinetic energy.
The answer is C.

Question 7

STEP 1 = > What do you need to determine to solve the problem?
You need to determine what factors influence vapour pressure in a closed container.

STEP 2 = > What relevant data provided in this problem is necessary in order to answer the question?
You need to recall some general information to answer this question.

STEP 3 = > Use the relevant data to solve the question
The vapour pressure of a liquid in a closed container will depend on the temperature. As the temperature increases, the rate of evaporation increased, so, the vapour pressure increase. The correct answer is C.

Question 8

STEP 1 = > What do you need to determine to solve the problem?
You need to determine the effect of altitude on boiling point.

STEP 2 = > What relevant data provided in this problem is necessary in order to answer the question?
This question is mostly a recall and reasoning question.

STEP 3 = > Use the relevant data to solve the question
At altitude the atmospheric pressure is lower. Therefore, it takes less energy for water molecules to break away from the liquid phase and enter into the vapour phase. Therefore, the correct answer is A.

Question 9

STEP 1 = > what do you need to determine to solve the problem?
You need to determine which statement is false.

STEP 2 = > what relevant data provided in this problem is necessary in order to answer the question?
You are provided with a phase diagram. This diagram provides information regarding all phase changes for a substance.

STEP 3 = > Use the relevant data to solve the question
Let's examine the choices. A) The vapour pressure of a substance at a given temperature. This statement is true. The curve that lies between the liquid and gas phase transition represents the vapour pressure curve – it gives information regarding temperatures and

pressures necessary to go from liquid to gas phase and visa versa. B) The sublimation point of a substance at a given temperature. This is true. Sublimation is the process by which a substance goes directly from its solid phase to a gas phase. The section of the diagram that has a curve separating the gas and solid phase will provide this information. C) The temperature and pressure beyond which the substance exists only in the vapour phase. This is also true. This statement refers to the critical point; this will be the point on the diagram where the vapour curve ends. And finally D) the types of intermolecular forces present at a given temperature. This statement is FALSE. While intermolecular forces will have an effect on phase transitions, they have nothing to do with the phase diagram, so the correct answer is D.

Question 10

STEP 1 = > what do you need to determine to solve the problem?
You need to determine the mole fraction of glucose in the solution.

STEP 2 = > what relevant data provided in this problem is necessary in order to answer the question?
You are told that the vapour pressure of each component in a solution will be equal to the mole fraction x the pressure of the pure substance. The total vapour pressure will be the sum of its components. In addition, you are provided with the total vapour pressure and the vapour pressure of water.

STEP 3 = > Use the relevant data to solve the question

$P_{solution} = (X_{solvent}) P^{o}_{solvent}$ (given in the question)

$X_{solvent} = 1 - X_{solute}$, since these are the only two components in the mixture

Therefore, $P_{solution} = (1 - X_{solute}) P^{o}_{solvent}$

So,

23.8 torr $= (1 - X_{solute})$ 30.5 torr

$(1 - X_{solute}) = 23.5/30.5$

$(1 - X_{solute}) = 0.7803$

$X_{solute} = 0.7803 - 1$

$X_{solute} = -0.2196$ $X_{solute} = 0.2196$

Mole fraction of glucose = 0.2196 – the correct answer is B.

Chapter 7: **Acids and Bases**

> *Tip:* **This is a common GAMSAT topic. It would be wise to understand the quick facts thoroughly as you may need them at RECALL level.**

Key Concept: Acids and Bases

There are a number of different definitions of acids and bases. In 1884, Svante Arrhenius defined an acid as a material that can release a proton or hydrogen ion. For instance, hydrogen chloride (HCl) in water ionized and becomes hydrogen ions and chloride ions. He defined a base as a material that can donate a hydroxide ion (OH^-). For example, sodium hydroxide (NaOH) in water becomes sodium ions and hydroxide ions. In 1923 Thomas Lowry altered this definition saying an acid can donate a proton and a base can accept a proton. G.N. Lewis made an even broader definition of acids and bases than Lowry in 1923. By his definitions, acids are electron pair acceptors and bases are electron pair donors.

The properties of acids and bases (based on the Arrhenius definitions) are as follows.

Properties of Acids
- Release hydrogen ion into water
- Neutralize bases in a neutralization reaction
- Corrode active metals
- Turn blue litmus to red
- Taste sour

Properties of Bases
- Release a hydroxide ion
- Neutralize acids in a neutralization reaction
- Denature proteins
- Turn red litmus blue
- Taste bitter

There are certain common acids and bases that are almost 100% ionized and these are called strong acids and bases. Weak acids and bases are incompletely ionized.

Common strong acids are
HNO_3 – nitric acids
HCl – hydrochloric acid
H_2SO_4 – sulphuric acid
$HClO_4$ – perchloric acid
HBr – hydrobromic acid
HI – hydroiodic acid

Of this list, only sulphuric aid is diprotic, meaning it has two ionisable hydrogens per formula. The other acids in this list are monoprotic because they have only one ionisable proton per formula. An acid with three ionisable protons would be triprotic, and any acid with 2 or more ionisable protons is called polyprotic.

Common strong bases
$LiOH$ – lithium hydroxide
$NaOH$ – sodium hydroxide
KOH – potassium hydroxide
$RbOH$ – rubidium hydroxide
$CsOH$ – cesium hydroxide
$Mg(OH)_2$ – magnesium hydroxide
$Ca(OH)_2$ – Calcium hydroxide
$Sr(OH)_2$ – strontium hydroxide
$Ba(OH)_2$ – barium hydroxide

The bases of the Group I metals are monobasic, the bases of the Group II metals are dibasic, bases with 3 ionisable hydroxyl group would be called tribasic, and those with 2 or more ionisable hydroxyl groups are called polybasic. Most of the alkaline organic compounds have an amino group ($-NH_2$) rather than an ionisable hydroxyl group. Since the amino group readily accepts a proton ($-NH_3$)$^+$, it definitely acts as a base according to the Lowry definition.

Note: It is always useful to memorize the strong acids and bases.

--->Quick facts: Acid Base Equilibrium

- A Bronsted-Lowry acid is a proton donor, while a Bronsted-Lowry base is a proton acceptor. When a Bronsted-Lowry acid donates its proton, it becomes a conjugate base and when the Bronsted-Lowry base accepts the proton, it becomes a conjugate acid.
- $[H_3O^+][OH^-]$ is said as the ionic product of water, the symbol is K_W. The value of it is constant in any aqueous solution, equals to 1.0×10^{-14}.
- $pH = -\log_{10}[H_3O^+(aq)]$

The pH value of a solution can be measured by using a pH meter and by using an indicator.

- For an acid HA, its acid dissociation constant (K_a) is: $[H^+(aq)][A^-(aq)] / [HA(aq)]$
- For a larger value of K_a, the acid is stronger, also the stronger the acid, the weaker its conjugate base.
- For a base B, its base dissociation constant (K_b) is:
- $[BH^+(aq)][OH^-] / [B(aq)]$
- For a larger value of K_b, the base is stronger, also, the stronger the base, the weaker its conjugate acid.
- $K_w = (K_a)(K_b)$
- A Lewis acid is an electric pair acceptor; a Lewis base is an electron pair donor. This is a broader definition.

Acid Strength is dependant on the following:

- The size of the atom to which the proton is attached; the larger the size of the atom, the stronger the acid.
  - The larger the atom the greater its surface area will be. The negative charge can be dispersed over the larger surface area stabilizing it. The more stabilized the anion, the less likely it will react with the hydrogen ion to reverse the process. In general if we compare acids with the other atoms are in the same group of the periodic table, the further down in the group the atom is, the stronger the acid will be.
  - $HI > HBr > HCl > HF$
  - $H_2S > H_2O$
- The electronegativity of the atom to which the proton is attached; the greater the electronegativity of the atom, the stronger the acid.
  - If we compare acid strength with acids where the atoms bonded to hydrogen were in the same period (same row in the periodic table), the difference in the size of the atoms would not be significant. In that case the electronegativity becomes the deciding factor.
  - $HF > H_2O > NH_3 > CH_4$

-     o $HCl > H_2S > PH_3 > SiH_4$
-     o   In addition, for MOST oxalic acids containing different elements in the same oxidation state from the same family acid, acid strength increases with increasing central element electronegativity.
-     o $HBrO_4 < HClO_4$
- The oxidation number of the central atom in molecule; the higher the oxidation number of the atom, the stronger the acid.
  -     o $HClO_4$ is a stronger acid than $HClO_3$ is a stronger acid than $HClO_2$ is a stronger acid than $HClO$.

Practice Questions: Acid Strength

Question 1-4

1. H_2SO_4 is a stronger acid than H_2SO_3 because
   i. it contains more oxygen attached to S than H_2SO_3
   ii. S has an oxidation state higher than the oxidation state of S in H_2SO_3
   iii. it has a higher molar mass than H_2SO_3

   A. I and II only
   B. I, II and III
   C. III only
   D. I only

2. The correct order of acidic strength is
   A. $HIO_4 > HBrO_4 > HClO_4$
   B. $HClO_4 > HBrO_4 > HIO_4$
   C. $HBrO_4 > HIO_4 > HClO_4$
   D. $HBrO_4 > HClO_4 > HIO_4$

3. The correct order of acidic strength is
   A. $HF < HCl < HI < HBr$
   B. $HI < HBr < HCl < HF$
   C. $HI < HBr < HF < HCl$
   D. $HF < HCl < HBr < HI$

4. In which of the following reaction is the italicized substance NOT acting as an acid?

A. $NaH(s)$ + $H_2O(l)$ → $H_2(g)$ + $Na^+(aq)$ + $OH^-(aq)$

B. $Mg_3N_2(s)$ + $6H_2O(l)$ → $3Mg(OH)_2(s)$ + $2NH_3(g)$

C. $HSO_4^-(aq)$ + $NH_3(g)$ → $NH_4^+(aq)$ + $SO_4^{2-}(aq)$

D. $NH_4^+(aq)$ + $NaNH_2(s)$ → $Na^+(aq)$ + $2NH_3(g)$

Solutions

Question 1-4

1. In the families of oxo acids, the greater the number of oxygen atoms attached to the central atom, the stronger the atom, and the stronger the acid. The statement (I) is correct. Also, the greater the oxidation state of the central atom, the stronger the acid.

Structure	Oxidation state
H_2SO_4	6
H_2SO_3	4

The correct answer is A.

2. The strongest acid is $HClO_4$; the strength of the acid depends on electronegativity in the case of oxalic acids. In terms of electronegativity, Cl > Br > I, so the answer is B.

3. The strength of an acid depends on a number of factors, in this case, the size of the atom is the major factor. Recall that the size of the atom within a group increases with increasing atomic mass. Therefore, the correct order is HF<HCl<HBr<HI, answer D.

4. In B, C and D the highlighted substance donates protons to a molecule contained in the second substance. In these three cases the named substance acts as an acid. The named substance in A, sodium hydride (or hydride ions), which has accepted a proton from water, is the base, and water is the acid. The simplified form of the equation is $H^- + H_2O → H_2 + OH^-$, the answer is A.

Key Concepts: Buffers and Indicators for Titrations

A buffer solution is a solution that can resist the pH change when a small amount of strong acid or alkali is added to it. A buffer solution is made by mixing a weak acid with its conjugate base, or a weak alkaline with its conjugate acid.

When a strong acid is added into a buffer solution, the conjugate base in the buffer will accept protons, to restore the pH. When a strong alkali is added, the weak acid in the buffer will neutralise the alkali, restoring the pH.

In order to determine the equivalence point of an acid-base titration accurately; a pH meter can be used through the process of titration. Any change in the pH of the solution can be recorded continuously. Then, by plotting a graph, the equivalence point can be determined more accurately. In GAMSAT you may be given a graph and questions related to the equivalence point.

Titrations can be classified into four kinds, they are: strong base -strong acid, strong base - weak acid, strong acid – weak base and weak acid – weak base.

The features of the above four titrations are shown in the following table. Study the table very carefully. (Refer below)

	strong base – strong acid	strong base – weak acid	strong acid – weak base	weak acid – weak base
Location of equivalence point	At pH value equals to 7 on the graph	At the alkaline part of the graph	At the acidic part of the graph	Cannot be detected
Location of steep portion on curve	Across almost the whole pH range	At the alkaline part of the graph	At the acidic part of the graph	No obvious steep portion
pH after the equivalence point is reached	Normally equal to 7	Larger than 7	Below 7	Normally equal to 7
Suitable indicator	Any indicator	Phenolphthalein	Methyl orange	No suitable indicator

An acid – base indicator is a substance that changes its colour when the pH of its environment changes. It changes its colour by changing its form to ionized or unionized. To choose an indicator, we want the indicator end point and the titration equivalence point close to each other. In order to determine the pH range of an indicator that will change its colour extremely, the relationship pK_a can be used.

To titrate soluble carbonates, a method of double indicator is used. The neutralizing process is divided into two parts. Consider K_2CO_3 as an example.
- Part 1: K_2CO_3 (aq) + HCl (aq) → $KHCO_3$ (aq) + KCl (aq)
- Part 2: $KHCO_3$ (aq) + HCl (aq) → KCl (aq) + H_2O (l) + CO_2 (g)

The end point of part 1 is indicated by phenolphthalein and part 2 is indicated by methyl orange, since the product solution in part 1 is alkaline and the product solution in part 2 is acidic.

In order to find the end point in weak acid – weak base titrations; the method of checking the conductivity of the solution is used. When the equivalence point is reached, the solution will have the highest conductivity, since the concentration of ions is maximized.

Figure 1 below illustrates the starting, end and equivalence points of various solutions.

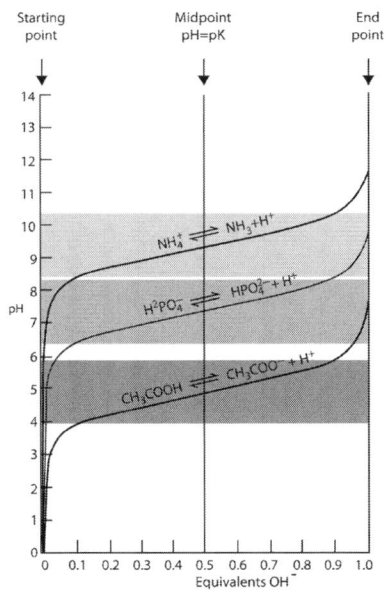

Figure 1

–->*Quick Facts: Buffers and Titration*

Buffers
- A buffer is a solution that resists changes in pH
- Can make a buffer with a weak acid and soluble salt containing the conjugate base OR a weak base and a soluble salt containing the conjugate acid
- Buffer is most effective in solutions where pH is at or close to the pKa of the weak acid
- In buffer solutions, the concentration of hydrogen ion IS NOT equal to the concentration of the conjugate ion
- There are four correct ways of writing the Henderson-Hasselbalch equation

  - $$pH = pKa - \log\frac{[HA]}{[A^-]}$$

  - $$pH = pKa + \log\frac{[A^-]}{[HA]}$$

  - $$pOH = pKb + \log\frac{[conjugate\_cation]}{[base]}$$

  - $$pOH = pKb - \log\frac{[base]}{[conjugate\_cation]}$$

- Equimolar buffer – equal concentrations of the weak acid (or base) and the conjugate ion

Titration
- Finding the concentration of an unknown liquid by comparing it to a known liquid
- A measured amount of the unknown material is mixed with an indicator and the known liquid
- The endpoint of the titration is shown by some types of indicator
- A pH indicator is usually one color above a characteristic pH and another colour below that pH

Practice Questions: pH

pH of a solution is defined as pH= -log $[H_3O^+]$

Also,

Ionic product of water, Kw = $[H_3O^+]$ $[OH^-]$

Questions 1-5

1. 4 g of caustic soda is dissolved in one litre solution, what will be the pH of the solution?

    A. 1.0
    B. 4.0
    C. 12.0
    D. 13.0

2. 2 M solutions of H_2SO_4 would have how many moles of H^+ ion in one litre?

    A. 1.0
    B. 2.0
    C. 3.0
    D. 4.0

3. What is the pH of a solution in which the $[OH^-]=1.0\times 10^{-4}$ M?

    A. 4.0
    B. 14
    C. 10
    D. +7

4. The pH of a neutral solution at 100°C when Kw = 1.0×10^{-12} is

    A. 7
    B. 6
    C. 0
    D. 12

5. The hydronium ion concentration in a neutral 0.00005 M $Ba(OH)_2$ solution is

   A. 10^{-4} M

   B. 10

   C. 10^{-10}

   D. 5×10^{-5}

Questions 6-9

6. An acid solution of pH 6 is diluted a hundred times. The pH of the solution becomes

   A. 6.95

   B. 6

   C. 4

   D. 8

7. If 0.36g of hydrogen chloride is dissolved to make a 1 litre solution (Cl=35.5 and H= 1), the pH concentration of the solution is

   A. 0.001

   B. 0.01

   C. 1.0

   D. 2.0

8. Given 0.200 M solution each of NH_4NO_3, $NaNO_3$ and Na_2CO_3. The correct order of increasing pH is

   A. $NH_4NO_3 < Na_2CO_3 < NaNO_3$

   B. $NH_4NO_3 < NaNO_3 < Na_2CO_3$

   C. $Na_2CO_3 < NaNO_3 < NH_4NO_3$

   D. $NaNO_3 < NH_4NO_3 < Na_2CO_3$

9. What is the pH of a 0.080 M CH_3COOH solution that is 4% dissociated?

   A. 2.92

   B. 0.80

   C. 2.49

   D. 5.26

Questions 10–11

10. The pH of 0.20 M HCOOH is between (Ka(HCOOH)=1.8×10^{-4})

    A. 2.0 and 2.5

    B. 2.5 and 3.0

    C. 3.0 and 3.5

    D. 3.5 and 4.0

11. What is the pH of a solution prepared by dissolving 0.100 mol of NaOH and 0.100 mol of HCl in enough water to make 1 L?

    A. 14.0

    B. 13.0

    C. 11.0

    D. 7.0

Solution

1. $[OH^-]=[NaOH]= \dfrac{\frac{4g}{40g/mol}}{1L} = 0.1M$

    $p[OH] = -\log[OH^-] = \log (0.1) = 1$

    $pH = 14 - p[OH] = 13$, answer D.

2. 1 mol H_2SO_4 in 1 L = 2 mol H^+ in 1 L .

    $\therefore 2$ mol H_2SO_4 in 1 L will furnish 4 moles H^+ ions in 1 L. The answer is D.

3. $[OH^-] = 1 \times 10^{-4}$ M

    $\therefore p[OH] = 4$

    and $pH = 14 - p[OH] = 10$, answer C.

4. $Kw = [H_3O^+]^2 = 1.0 \times 10^{-12}$

    $\therefore [H_3O^+] = 1.0 \times 10^{-6}$

    $pH = -\log (1.0 \times 10^{-6})$

    $= 6$, the answer is B.

5. 1 mol $Ba(OH)_2$ = 2 mol (OH^-)

$\therefore [OH^-]$ = 2 × 0.00005 M

because the solution is neutral, $[H_3O^+]$ = $[OH^-]$ = 1.0×10^{-4} M

The correct answer is A.

6. pH=6

$[H_3O^+]$ = 10^{-6} M

When the solution is diluted 100 times then new acid concentration becomes 10^{-8} M. Now H_3O^+ contribution from the ionization of water cannot be ignored. Therefore

$[H_3O^+]$ = 10^{-8} M (from acid) + 10^{-7} (from H_2O) = 1.1×10^{-7}

$\therefore$ pH = -log (1.1×10^{-7}) = 6.95, answer A.

7. $[H^+]=[HCl]= \dfrac{\frac{0.36g}{36.5g/mol}}{1l} = 0.01M$

pH = -log$[H^+]$ = -log (0.01) = 2

pH = 2, answer D.

8. Examining the different salts and their dissociation in water you have:

NH_4NO_3 will form nitric acid and ammonia.

$NaNO_3$ will form nitric acid and sodium hydroxide.

Na_2CO_3 will form carbonic acid and sodium hydroxide..

Now examine the strengths of the acid and base in each pair. Ammonia is a relatively weak base, while nitric acid is a strong acid, this will make the overall pH of NH_4NO_3 acidic. In the case of $NaNO_3$ you have both a strong acid and a strong base, so the pH will be closed to neutral. Finally, carbonic acid is a weaker acid than nitric acid since C is less electronegative than N. So the pH of Na_2CO_3 will be higher than $NaNO_{3.}$ Therefore, the correct order is given in answer B.

9. From the ionization of acetic acid,

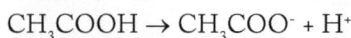

$CH_3COOH \rightarrow CH_3COO^- + H^+$

$[CH_3COOH]$ = 0.08M

$[CH_3COO^-]$ = $[H^+]$ = 4% × 0.08 = 0.0032

pH = -log(0.0032) = 2.49; answer C.

10. You are told that you have a 0.2M solution of HCOOH and given the Ka. You know

that $K_a = \dfrac{[H^+][HCOO^-]}{[HCOOH]}$. At the start of the reaction you have 0.2M formic acid

and no H^+ or $HCOO^-$. After some time, there will be 0.2-x formic acid left and
x of each of the other two components formed. So you now have

$1.8 \times 10^{-4} = \dfrac{x^2}{(0.2-x)}$. Since x will be << less than 0.2 you can assume that

$1.8 \times 10^{-4} = \dfrac{x^2}{0.2}; x = 0.006$

$pH = -\log[H^+] = -\log[0.006] = 2.22$

The answer is A.

11. You are making a buffer from a strong acid and a strong base. In this case, the pH will
equal 7 since they will neutralize each other. Therefore the answer is D.

Key Concepts: Acid-Base Indicators

How do acid-base indicator works?

Acid-base indicators work by marking the end point of a titration by changing colour. The most
common acid-base indicators are complex molecules that are themselves weak acids. They exhibit
one colour when the proton is attached to the molecule and a different colour when the proton
is absent. For example, phenolphthalein, a commonly used indicator is colourless in its HIn
form and pink in its In⁻ or basic form. To see how molecules such as phenolphthalein function
as indicators, consider the following equilibrium for some hypothetical indicator HIn of a weak
acid with $K_a = 1.0 \times 10^{-8}$.

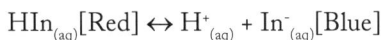

$$HIn_{(aq)}[Red] \leftrightarrow H^+_{(aq)} + In^-_{(aq)}[Blue]$$

$$K_a = \frac{[H^+][In^-]}{[HIn]}$$

$$\frac{K_a}{[H^+]} = \frac{[In^-]}{[HIn]}$$

Suppose we add a few drops of this indicator to an acidic solution whose pH is 1.0 ($[H^+]$ = 1.0 × 10^{-1}). Then

$$\frac{K_a}{[H^+]} = \frac{[1.0 \times 10^{-8}]}{[1.0 \times 10^{-1}]} = 10^{-7} = \frac{1}{10,000,000} = \frac{[In^-]}{[HIn]}$$

This ratio shows that the predominant form of the indicator is HIn, resulting in a red solution. As OH^- is added to this solution in a titration, $[H^+]$ decreases and the equilibrium shifts to the right, changing HIn to In^-. At some point in a titration, enough of the In^- form will be present in the solution so that a purple tint will be noticeable. That is, a colour change from red to reddish purple will occur. We will assume, then, that in the titration of acid with a base, the colour change will occur at a pH where

$$\frac{[In^-]}{[HIn]} = \frac{1}{10}$$

How to determine an appropriate indicator for a titration, given the equivalence point of the titration and K_a (or pK_a) values for possible indicators.

Just choose an indicator whose pKa value falls around the equivalence point of the titration.
The importance of pK_{ind}
Think about a general indicator, HInd - where "Ind" is all the rest of the indicators apart from the hydrogen ion which is given away:

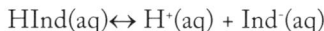

$$HInd(aq) \leftrightarrow H^+(aq) + Ind^-(aq)$$

Because this is just like any other weak acid, you can write an expression for K_a for it. We will call it K_{ind} to stress that we are talking about the indicator.

$$K_{Ind} = \frac{[H^+][Ind^-]}{[HInd]}$$

Think of what happens half-way through the colour change. At this point the concentrations of the acid and its ion are equal. In that case, they will cancel out of the K_{ind} expression.

$$K_{Ind} = \frac{[H^+][Ind^-]}{[HInd]}$$

$$K_{Ind} = [H^+]$$

Figure 2 shows the equivalence points and thus the colour change of both methyl orange and phenolphthalein indicators.

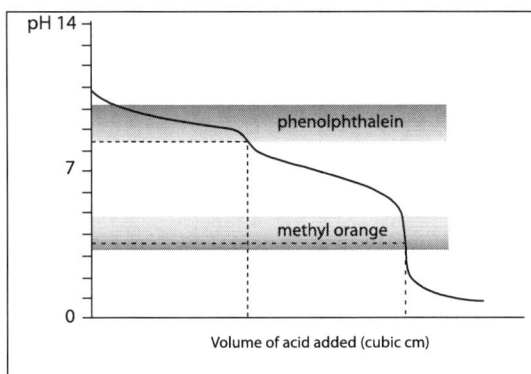

Figure 2

Practice QUESTIONS

Question 1-4

Some of the common indicators used in titration are given in the table on the next page. The acid base titration curves of 1-L solutions of 1 M acetic acid, $H_2PO_4^-$ and NH_4^+ by strong base are shown in Figure 2. The curves have similar shape, but are shifted vertically along the pH axis. The slope of each titration curve is much lesser near its midpoint than it is near its wings.

pK_a values are given below
acetic acid – 4.76
$H_2PO_4^-$ – 7.20
NH_4^+ – 9.25

Name	Acid Colour	pH Range of Colour Change	Base Colour
Methyl violet	Yellow	0.0 - 1.6	Blue
Thymol blue	Red	1.2 - 2.8	Yellow
Methyl orange	Red	3.2 - 4.4	Yellow
Bromocresol green	Yellow	3.8 - 5.4	Blue
Methyl red	Red	4.8 - 6.0	Yellow
Litmus	Red	5.0 - 8.0	Blue
Bromothymol blue	Yellow	6.0 - 7.6	Blue
Thymol blue	Yellow	8.0 - 9.6	Blue
Phenolphthalein	Colourless	8.2 - 10.0	Pink
Thymolphthalein	Colourless	9.4 - 10.6	Blue
Alizarin yellow R	Yellow	10.1 – 12.0	Red

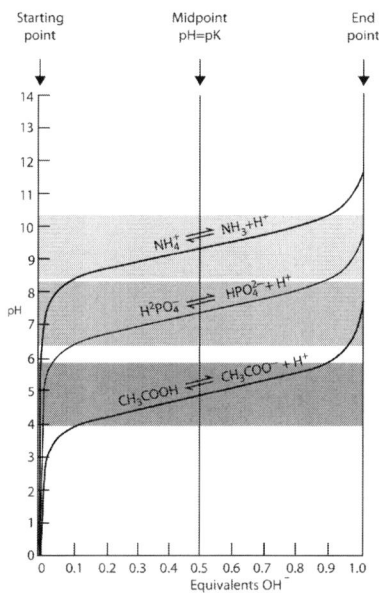

1. For all the solutions, the pH at the point where the equivalents of OH⁻ added is equal to the equivalent of acid initially present,

    A. is equal to seven

    B. is equal to 0.5

    C. is greater than seven

    D. is less than seven, but not equal to 0.5

2. The pH of the solution is relatively insensitive to the addition of the strong base or strong acid at the

    A. starting point

    B. mid point

    C. end point

    D. nowhere

3. $H_2PO_4^-$ is in its useful buffer range, when

    A. pH > 9.8

    B. pH < 2.8

    C. 6.3 < pH < 8.3

    D. only when pH is equal to 10

4. Referring to the table and figure, Phenolphthalein can be effectively used at each of it's three equivalence point for detecting the strong base for

    A. acetic acid

    B. NH_4Cl

    C. H_3PO_4

    D. all of them

Question 5-8

A conjugate acid is a Bronsted-acid formed when Bronsted base has accepted a proton. A conjugate base is a Bronsted base formed when a Bronsted acid donates proton.

5. The conjugate acid of HPO_4^{2-} is

    A. PO_4^{3-}

    B. $H_2PO_4^-$

    C. H_3PO_3

    D. PO_3^{3-}

6. The conjugate base of H_2S is
   - A. S^{2-}
   - B. H_2S
   - C. HS^-
   - D. H_2S_4

7. The conjugate base of $N_2H_5^+$ is
   - A. N_2H_4
   - B. $N_2H_4^+$
   - C. $N_2H_4^-$
   - D. N_2H_6

8. In the equilibrium reaction
   $$CH_3COOH + HF \leftrightarrow CH_3COOH_2^{\oplus} + F^-$$
   - A. F^- is the conjugate acid of HF
   - B. F^- is the conjugate base of HF
   - C. F^- is the conjugate acid of CH_3COOH
   - D. $CH_3COOH_2^{\oplus}$ is the conjugate base of CH_3COOH

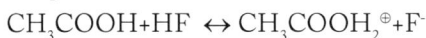

Solution

Question 1-8

1. pH at the equivalence point is > 7 because of the reaction of A^- with H_2O to form HA + OH^-, The answer is C.

2. When HA = A^-, the pH of the solution is relatively insensitive to the addition of strong base or strong acid B.

3. A weak acid is in the useful buffer range when pH= pKa + or − 1
   Hence the answer is C.

4. Phenolphthalein can be used in the range of 8.2 and 10. Hence answer is B.

5. A conjugate acid is a Bronsted- acid formed when Bronsted base has accepted a proton. When HPO_4^{2-} accepts a proton, it forms $H_2PO_4^-$, which is a conjugate acid of HPO_4^{2-}. This is given in answer B.

6. A conjugate base is a Bronsted base formed when a Bronsted acid donates proton. Bronsted acid $- H^+ \rightarrow$ conjugate base HS^- is a conjugate base of Bronsted acid H_2S, answer C.

7. The conjugate base of $N_2H_5^+$ is N_2H_4, answer A.

8. In the reaction
$$CH_3COOH + HF \leftrightarrow CH_3COOH_2^\oplus + F$$

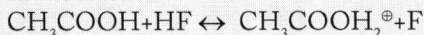

HF has donated a proton to CH_3COOH and itself converted into F^-. Therefore, F^- is a conjugate base of HF; answer B.

GAMSAT Style Questions

Questions 1-4

The body has a wide array of mechanisms to maintain homeostasis in the blood and extracellular fluid. The most important way that the pH of the blood is kept relatively constant is by buffers dissolved in the blood. The body maintains the blood pH at 7.4, as even a few tenths of a change in pH can result in serious health complications. The pH of a buffer system can be calculated using the Henderson-Hasselbach equation which says that pH = pK_a + log ([conjugate base]/[conjugate acid]). By far, the most important buffer for maintaining acid-base balance in the blood is the carbonic acid-bicarbonate buffer.

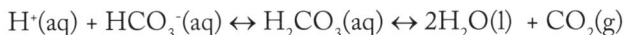

$$H^+(aq) + HCO_3^-(aq) \leftrightarrow H_2CO_3(aq) \leftrightarrow 2H_2O(l) + CO_2(g)$$

1. If a base was added to this buffer system, which molecule would it react with it in the above equation to prevent a change in pH?

   A. HCO_3^-
   B. CO_2
   C. H_2O
   D. H_2CO_3

2. The dissociated bicarbonate ion is the predominant species over carbonic acid. If the ratio of bicarbonate ion to carbonic acid in the body is 10:1. What information does this give about the pKa of the acid in this system?

   A. pK_a is 5.4
   B. pK_a is 6.4
   C. pK_a is 7.4
   D. pK_a is 8.4

3. Without this buffer system, certain activities would alter the pH balance within the blood. Metabolism that results in proton production. Exhalation results in the loss of CO_2 and water. What effect might each of these have on the pH of blood?

   A. Metabolism could cause a decrease in pH/ exhalation could cause a decrease in pH

   B. Metabolism could cause an increase in pH/ exhalation could cause an increase in pH

   C. Metabolism could cause a decrease in pH/ exhalation could cause an increase in pH

   D. Metabolism could cause a decrease in pH/ exhalation could cause a decrease in pH

4. Another buffer system present in the body is the phosphate buffer system present in the internal fluid of all cells:

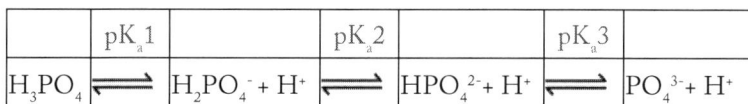

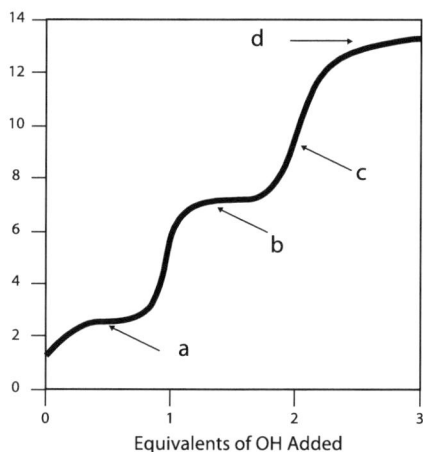

	pK_a1		pK_a2		pK_a3	
H_3PO_4 ⇌		$H_2PO_4^- + H^+$ ⇌		$HPO_4^{2-} + H^+$ ⇌		$PO_4^{3-} + H^+$

Equivalents of OH Added

Which letter is pointing to the point on the titration curved where the buffering range is most effective in the cells of the body?

A. B

B. D

C. C

D. A

Solution

Question 1

STEP 1 = > What do you need to determine to solve the problem?
Which molecule in the buffer reaction would interact with a base.

STEP 2 = > What relevant data provided in this problem is necessary in order to answer the question?
You are given the buffer reaction, and therefore can determine which molecules act as the proton donors and proton acceptors to create the buffer system that prevents a drastic change in pH.

STEP 3 = > Use the relevant data to solve the question
To answer this problem, you need to understand how a buffer prevents changes in pH. It contains an acid/base pair that can react with either excess acid or base that may be added into the system to prevent any changes in pH. To neutralize any added base, the molecule acting as the acid will react with it. In this case, the H_2CO_3 has the extra proton available to react with a base, thus the answer is D.

Question 2

STEP 1 = > What do you need to determine to solve the problem?
The relationship of the pKa of carbonic acid to the pH of blood.

STEP 2 = > What relevant data provided in this problem is necessary in order to answer the question?
As for the previous problem, you are given the buffer reaction. In addition you are told that the ratio of bicarbonate to carbonic acid is about 10:1. Finally, the passage gives you the equation necessary to calculate pK_a using pH and the concentrations of base and acid in the system.

STEP 3 = > Use the relevant data to solve the question
Use the Henderson-Hasselbach equation which states that pH = pK_a + log ([conjugate base]/[conjugate acid]). Thus pK_a = pH – log ([conjugate base]/[conjugate acid]). Now, you simply need to determine which species is the acid and which is the base. In this case, the carbonic acid has the extra proton that it can donate so it is acting as the acid. The bicarbonate, with its negative charge can accept a proton, so it is acting as the base. Therefore, you know that the pK_a = 7.4 – log(10). Since log(10) = 1, the pK_a must be lower than the pH by a value of 1, thus the answer is 6.4, B.

Question 3

STEP 1 = > What do you need to determine to solve the problem?
You need to determine how metabolism and exhalation can affect blood pH.

STEP 2 = > What relevant data provided in this problem is necessary in order to answer the question?
You are given the reaction showing that bicarbonate will acquire a proton to produce carbonic acid. In addition, the carbonic acid breaks down to carbon dioxide and water. These processes are normally at equilibrium in the body. You are told that metabolism produces more protons, and exhalation results in the loss of carbon dioxide and water.

STEP 3 = > Use the relevant data to solve the question:
Examining the reaction allows you to determine the effect that each process will have on it. Excess H^+ will shift the first part of the reaction to the right, and therefore more acid will be formed. Thus, the additional H^+ will cause the blood pH to be lower than 7.4. On the other hand, the loss of CO_2 and water that result from respiration will cause the second part of the reaction to shift to the right. In this case, more carbonic acid will break down to make up for the lost CO_2 and water and return the system to an equilibrium state. The loss of carbonic would result in more basic conditions and thus an increase in the pH. Therefore, the answer is C.

Question 4

STEP 1 = > What do you need to determine to solve the problem?
You need to determine the point on the titration curve where the buffer would be most effective in a cell.

STEP 2 = > What relevant data provided in this problem is necessary in order to answer the question?
You are given the reaction equation for the phosphate buffer and a graphical representation of the titration curve. The curve shows three points with a very shallow slope, indicating three different equivalence points. The equation shows three reactions in equilibrium with a different pK_a for each.

STEP 3 = > Use the relevant data to solve the question
From the original passage, you know the pH of the blood is 7.4. From this, you can deduce that pH in most body systems should be approximately 7. The question is asking for where the buffering range is most effective, or where there will be the least change in pH with the addition of acid or base. In graphical terms, this means where the slope is close to 0. This occurs at points a, b, and d. So, how do you decide which point would be best for buffering in cells? As mentioned, the pH of most systems in the body will be around 7. A buffer will be most effective when the pK_a is close to the pH. Therefore, the answer is A-point b.

Chapter 8: **Electrochemistry**

> *Tip:* This topic is also a favourite for the GAMSAT. Study the quick facts well, do the questions because once you understand the questions this is easy marks.

Key Concepts: Electrolytic Cells

Electrochemistry is the study of the changes that cause electrons to flow, creating what we call electricity. This flow of electrons is created by reduction and oxidation reactions (redox). Redox reactions were discussed previously in Chapter 2.

When electricity is passed through a liquid solution of an ion or an electrolyte, a chemical reaction called *electrolysis* occurs. When electricity flows, chemical changes happen. For example, let's take a solution of sodium chloride. At the positive electrode, the *anode*, oxidation occurs as electrons are pulled from negatively charged chloride ions.

$$2Cl^- \rightarrow Cl_2 + 2e^-$$

At the negative electrode, the *cathode*, reduction occurs as electrons are added to positively charged sodium ions.

$$Na^+ + e^- \rightarrow Na$$

In affect, it splits the sodium and chlorine back into their elements.

Remember the anode is where oxidation occurs (remember "an ox"). The cathode is where reduction occurs (remember "red cat").

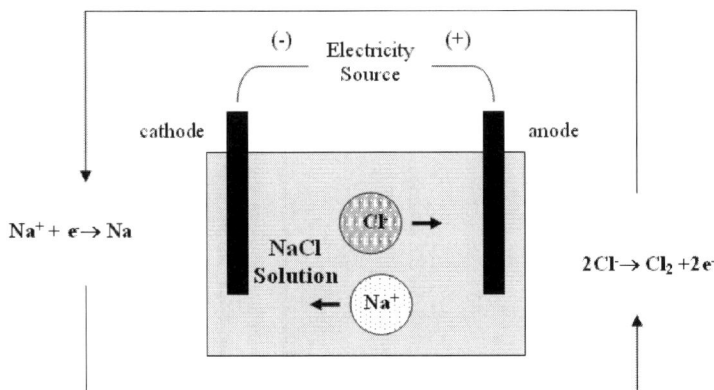

In electrolytic cells, the redox reaction is non-spontaneous and needs electrical energy to induce electrolysis.

Key Concepts: Galvanic Cells

Galvanic cells, also known as voltaic cells, are basically batteries. In this type of cell, the redox reaction is spontaneous.

If we place a piece of copper into a silver nitrate solution, a spontaneous reaction occurs. The solution turns blue due to the formation of copper (II) nitrate and a greyish white silver deposit forms on the piece of copper.

$$2Ag^+ + Cu \rightarrow Cu^{2+} + 2Ag$$

However, no usable energy can be acquired from this reaction because it is released and dissipated as heat. Now, if this same chemical reaction is placed into a galvanic cell, it can produce electricity. A galvanic cell consists of two containers with a salt bridge between them. Each container stores one of the half reactions of a redox reaction. Lets again consider the above reaction, but divide it into two half reactions.

$$\text{Oxidation: } Cu \rightarrow Cu^{2+} + 2e^-$$
$$\text{Reduction: } Ag^+ + 2e^- \rightarrow Ag$$

In a galvanic cell, each half reaction is contained in two separate containers and they remain electrically neutral. The salt bridge allows ions to enter and leave the solutions.

The electron flow from the anode to the cathode is what creates electricity. In a galvanic cell, the cathode is positive and the anode is negative, while in an electrolytic cell, the opposite occurs.

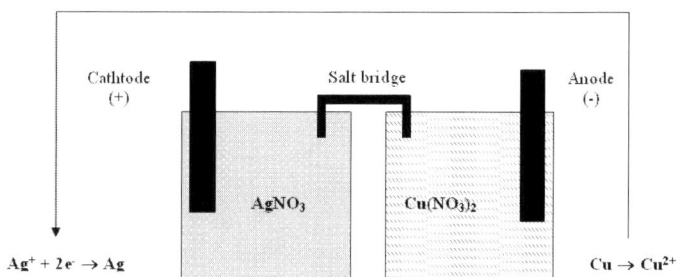

The conventional way of representing an electrochemical cell of any kind is to write the oxidation half reaction on the left and the reduction on the right. Thus, for the reaction

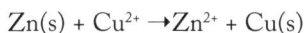

$Zn(s) + Cu^{2+} \rightarrow Zn^{2+} + Cu(s)$

We write

$Zn(s) \mid Zn^{2+}(aq) \mid\mid Cu^{2+}(aq) \mid Cu(s)$

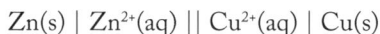

In which the single vertical bars represent *phase boundaries*. The double bar denotes a *liquid-liquid boundary*, which in laboratory cells consists of a salt bridge or in ion-permeable barrier. If the net cell reaction were written in reverse, the cell notation would become

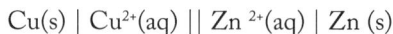

$Cu(s) \mid Cu^{2+}(aq) \mid\mid Zn^{2+}(aq) \mid Zn(s)$

Remember: the **Reduction** process is always shown on the **Right**.

The transfer of electrons between an electrode and the solution takes place by quantum-mechanical *tunnelling* at the electrode surface. The energy required to displace water molecules from the hydration shell of an ion as it approaches the electrode surface constitutes the *activation energy*. This can slow down the process. Even larger activation energies (and slower reactions) occur when a molecule such as O_2 is formed or consumed.

Key Concepts: Faraday's laws of electrolysis

The decomposition of an electrolyte by passing an electric current is called electrolysis.

The weight of an element liberated at a given electrode during electrolysis is directly proportional to the quantity of electricity passing through the electrolyte.

If W grams of an element are liberated from an electrolyte by passing a current of C amperes strength for t seconds through it,

Then, $W \propto C \times t$ (Quantity of electricity in coulombs = strength of the current in amperes × time in seconds for which it is passed, or **W = C × t × z**. Where z is the constant of proportionality in the above equation and is called the electro-chemical equivalent.

When C = 1 ampere, and t = 1 second (i.e. when a current of 1 ampere strength is passed through the electrolyte for one second), W = z.

Hence, the electro-chemical equivalent of an ion is its weight in grams that is liberated by one ampere-current in one second (i.e. by one coulomb of electricity).

The quantity of electricity involved in using a current of 1 ampere strength for one second is 1 coulomb (i.e. coulomb = ampere × second).

(ii) According the Faraday's law, the weight deposited at an electrode = (Current in amps) (time in sec) (GEW of substance deposited) / 96,500.

Important conversions:

1 Faraday = 96500 coulombs = 1 mole of e^-

1 C = 1 amp s

Practice Questions

1-Questions where you have to find out the current flowing through the cell.

Questions 1-6

SITUATION 1
Reduction reaction will be given. You have to deduce any of the parameters related using Faraday's Law.

The reduction reaction that occurs during the reduction of $Cr_2O_7^{2-}$ can be represented by the equation:
$Cr_2O_7^{2-}+6e^- +14H^+\rightarrow 2Cr^{3+} +7H_2O$

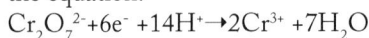

1. The number of coulombs required to reduce one mole of $Cr_2O_7^{2-}$ to Cr^{3+} is

    A. 96500C

    B. 9650 C

    C. 289500 C

    D. 579000 C

The reduction of one iron oxide to another can be represented by the equation:
$2Fe^{3+} + 2e^- \rightarrow 2Fe^{2+}$

2. One mole of iron (III) oxide can be reduced to iron (II) oxide by passing

    A. 1F

    B. 2F

    C. 3F

    D. 6F

SITUATION 2
Mass will be given. You have to deduce any of the parameters related using Faraday's Law.

3. If the molecular mass of nitrobenzene, $C_6H_5NO_2$, is 123, the number of coulombs required to reduce 12.3g of nitrobenzene to aniline $C_6H_5NH_2$ is

    A. 57900C

    B. 115800 C

    C. 28950 C

    D. 5790 C

SITUATION 3
The amount of substance formed at the cathode or anode will be given. You have to deduce any of the parameters related using Faraday's Law.

4. 0.112 L of O_2 at STP is collected at the anode in 965s.
   If the anode reaction is $2H_2O \rightarrow O_2 + 4e^- + 4H^+$
   The current in amperes passed through the cell is

   A. 2A

   B. 0.5 A

   C. 0.2 A

   D. 965 A

5. Calculate the current in amperes that must be passed for 965 s through a solution of $CuSO_4$ in order to deposit 1g of copper. (m.wt. of Cu = 64)

   A. 100 A

   B. 3.125 A

   C. 31.25 A

   D. 200 A

6. The number of electrons required to deposit 1g of aluminium from molten Al_2O_3 will be (m.wt. of Al = 27) N_A = Avogadro's number

   A. $1 \times N_A$

   B. $2 \times N_A$

   C. $0.11 \times N_A$

   D. $3 \times N_A$

2- Questions where you have to find out the quantity of the deposited material, time and other parameters.

7. A passage of 10A of current for 965 sec through acidified water results in the evolution of H_2 gas at the cathode. The amount of O_2 gas produced at the anode is

   A. 0.05 mol

   B. 0.05 g

   C. 0.025 mol

   D. 0.025 g

8. An electric current of 5A through copper sulfate solution increases the mass of the cathode by 32g. The time for which the current would have been passed is, (m.wt. Cu = 64)

    A. 193 sec

    B. 96.5 sec

    C. 19300 sec

    D. 96500 sec

Solution

1. The basic equation is given.

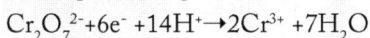

$$Cr_2O_7^{2-} + 6e^- + 14H^+ \rightarrow 2Cr^{3+} + 7H_2O$$

The reduction of one mole of $Cr_2O_7^{2-}$ to Cr^{3+} requires $6e^-$ and thus 6F.

6×96500 C = 579000 C. This is given in answer D.

2. One mole Fe_2O_3 can be reduced to FeO by passing a 2F of electricity since $2e^-$ are needed to reduce Fe^{3+} to Fe^{2+}.

$$2Fe^{3+} + 2e^- \rightarrow 2Fe^{2+}$$

The correct answer is B.

3. The molecular mass of nitrobenzene, $C_6H_5NO_2$, is 123 g/mol.

When nitrobenzene is converted to aniline nitrogen is reduced from +4 to -2 oxidation state. So in this reduction reaction nitrogen in +4 oxidation state gain 6 electrons and converted into -2 oxidation state.

The number of moles of nitrobenzene = $\dfrac{12.3}{123}$ = 0.1.

When 1 mole of nitrobenzene is reduced to aniline 6 moles of electrons are transferred.

0.1 moles nitrobenzene × 6 moles of electrons / 1 mole of nitrobenzene

= 0.6 moles of electrons

1 mole of electrons = 9.65×10^4 C

0.6 moles of electrons × 9.65×10^4 C / 1 mole of electron

= 57900 C

The correct answer is A.

4. First you need to calculate how many moles of O_2 you have in 0.112L of O_2.
You are told that you are at STP. At STP, P = 1 atm, T = 273K.
Using the ideal gas law equation $PV=nRT$ – remember R is a constant
$$R= 0.0821 \text{ L-atm/mol-K}$$
You get 1atm (0.112L) = n (0.0821 L-atm/mol-K) (273K)
$$n = 0.005 \text{ mol , weight of } O_2 \text{ collected at the anode} = 0.16g.$$
According the Faraday's Laws:
Weight deposited at an electrode = (Current in amps) (time in sec) (gram equivalent weight of substance deposited) / 96,500.
The gram equivalent weight = m.wt./ the mole of electron gained or lost per mole of substance being oxidized or reduced.

The anode reaction is

$2H_2O \rightarrow O_2 + 4e^- + 4H^+$

So, For O_2 GEW = $\frac{2(16)}{4} = 8$

0.16g O_2 = current (965) (8)/96500
Current = 2 amps
The answer is A.

5. $Cu^{2+} + 2e^- \rightarrow Cu(s)$

GEW of Cu = $\frac{64}{2}$ = 32

Weight deposited at an electrode = (Current in amps) (time in sec) (gram equivalent weight of substance deposited) / 96,500

1 g Cu = $\frac{current(965s)(32)}{96500}$

Current = 3.125 amps - the answer is B.

6. In Al_2O_3, the oxidation state of Al is +3. The reaction for the deposition of Al is
$2Al_2O_3(s) \rightarrow 4Al(s) + 3O_2(g)$
Recall that oxidation state of Al in Al_2O_3 will be 2x + (-2(3))=0; 2x = 6, so x=3 which is the oxidation state of Al.
So for aluminium, the half reaction is $Al^{3+} + 3e^- \rightarrow Al$
So for 1g Al = 0.037 moles of Al
There are 3 moles of electrons necessary for every 1 mole of Al, so for 1g of Al, 0.11 moles of e^- will be needed. To find the number of electrons remember that one mole of electrons = Avogadro's number, which you are told is N_A. So, the number of electrons will be 0.11 × N_A. The answer is C.

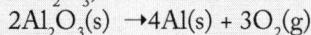

7. You are given the following values

    Current - 10A

    Time - 965 sec

According the Faraday's Laws:

Weight deposited at an electrode = (Current in amps) (time in sec) (gram equivalent weight of substance deposited) / 96,500

The reaction at the anode is

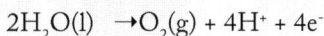

$2H_2O(l) \rightarrow O_2(g) + 4H^+ + 4e^-$

So amount of O2 $= \dfrac{10A(965s)\dfrac{32}{4}}{96500}$

$\qquad\qquad\quad = 0.8g$

that is, the mole of $O_2 = 0.025$ mol of O_2 – the answer is C.

8. You are given the following values:

Electric current of 5A

Mass of the element formed at the cathode - 32g

M.wt. Cu = 64g

According the Faraday's Laws: weight deposited at an electrode = (Current in amps) (time in sec) (gram equivalent weight of substance deposited) / 96,500

The reaction at the cathode

    $Cu^{2+} + 2e^- \rightarrow Cu$

So 32g Cu $= \dfrac{5A(t)(\dfrac{64}{2})}{96500}$

t = 19300 sec – the answer is C.

GAMSAT Style Questions

Question 1-2

Faraday's first law of electrolysis states, "The mass of an ion discharged during electrolysis is proportional to the quantity of electricity passed".

$M \propto Q$

$M \propto It$

$M = ZIt$ where I = current in amperes

                        t = time is seconds

and Z = electrochemical equivalent of the ion deposited and is defined as the mass of the ion deposited by passing a current of one ampere for one second. Its unit is gram per coulomb. According the Faraday's law, the weight deposited at an electrode = ($I \times t \times$ gram equivalent weight of the substance deposited) / 96,500.

1. One Faraday of electricity was passed through the electrolytic cells placed in series containing molten Al_2O_3, an aqueous solution of $CuSO_4$ and molten $NaCl$ respectively for 1 sec. The amount of Al, Cu and Na deposited at the cathode will be (m.wt, Al = 27; Cu = 64; Na = 23)

	Al	Cu	Na
A.	1/3 moles	1/2 mole	1 mole
B.	1 mole	2 moles	3 moles
C.	3 moles	1.5 moles	1 mole
D.	3 moles	2.5 moles	3 moles

2. A certain current liberated 5.64 L hydrogen gas in 7.200×10^3 s at STP. How many grams of Ni can be deposited by the same current flowing for the same time in a nickel sulfate solution (m.wt. of Ni = 59).

    A. 14.8g

    B. 29.74g

    C. 7.430g

    D. 0.01708g

Question 3-4

Exactly 0.200 mole electrons are passed through two electrolytic cells in series. One contains silver ion, and the other, zinc ion. Assume that the only cathode reaction in each cell is the reduction of the ion to the metal. The cathode reactions in the two electrolytic cells are

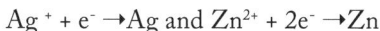

$$Ag^+ + e^- \rightarrow Ag \text{ and } Zn^{2+} + 2e^- \rightarrow Zn$$

3. How many g of each will be deposited? (m.wt: Zn= 65, Ag = 108)

    A. 108g Ag and 65g Zn

    B. 108g Ag and 32.5g Zn

    C. 21.6g Ag and 6.5g Zn

    D. 21.6g Ag and 13.0g Zn

4. A certain current liberates 0.504g hydrogen in 2.00 hours. How many grams of oxygen can be liberated by the same current in the same time?

    A. 4.00g O_2

    B. 8.00g O_2

    C. 16.0g O_2

    D. 32.0g O_2

Question 5

A current of 2.00 A passing for 1.93×10^4 s through a molten tin salt deposits 23.8g tin (at. Mass: 119). The oxidation state of the tin in the salt is:

    A. 2

    B. 4

    C. 1

    D. 3

Question 6-8

An electrolyte (AB) when dissolved in water or when melted dissociates to produce ions: $AB \rightarrow A^+ + B^-$. When the circuit is closed, the following reactions occur at the two electrodes:

    (a) The cations move towards the cathode and gain electrons. The battery pumps electrons into the cathode and reduction takes place.

    $A^+ + e^- \rightarrow A$ (reduction)

    (b) The battery pumps electrons out of the anode, and substances capable of being oxidized (anions) give electrons up at the anode.

    The cathode is the negative terminal during electrolysis and the anode is the positive terminal.

6. The oxidizing agent in the reaction

    $2MnO_4^- + 5C_2O_4^{2-} + 16H^+ \rightarrow 2Mn^{2+} + 10CO_2 + 8H_2O$ is:

    A. $C_2O_4^{2-}$ ion

    B. MnO_4^- ion

    C. H^+ ion

    D. All three ions

7. In the following reaction, the value of X is

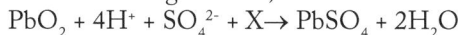

$PbO_2 + 4H^+ + SO_4^{2-} + X \rightarrow PbSO_4 + 2H_2O$

    A. $2e^-$

    B. $4e^-$

    C. $1e^-$

    D. $6e^-I$

8. In the reduction of gold from the $AuCl_4^-$ ion, the solution must be stirred rapidly during electrolysis. The stirring is important

    A. To separate gold from chlorine

    B. Because it increases the conductivity of the solution

    C. Because it increases the movement of $AuCl_4^-$ towards anode

    D. Because it overcomes the repulsion between the $AuCl_4^-$ and the excess electron at the electrode and helps in deposition of gold.

Question 9-11

    Given: $E^\circ_{Al^{3+}/Al} = -1.66$ V, $E^\circ_{Fe^{2+}/Fe} = -0.40$V, $E^\circ_{Cu^{2+}/Cu} = +0.34$ V, $E^\circ_{Mg^{2+}/Mg} = -2.37$ V

9. The metal salt solution that can be stored in the other three metal containers is:

    A. $MgSO_4$ solution

    B. $Al_2(SO_4)_3$ solution

    C. $FeSO_4$ solution

    D. $CuSO_4$ solution

10. The correct order of increasing reactivity is:

    A. Al<Cu<Fe<Mg

    B. Cu<Fe<Al<Mg

    C. Cu<Al<Mg<Fe

    D. Mg<Al<Fe<Cu

11. The strongest reducing agent is:

    A. Al

    B. Fe

    C. Cu

    D. Mg

Question 12

A 1 molar solution each of $Cu(NO_3)_2$, $Ag(NO_3)$, $Hg_2(NO_3)_2$, $Mg(NO_3)_2$ is being electrolyzed by using inert electrodes. The values of standard electrode potentials in volts are

$$E°_{Ag^+/Ag} = +0.80 \text{ V}, E°_{Hg_2^{2+}/Hg} = +0.79 \text{ V}, E°_{Mg^{2+}/Mg} = -2.37 \text{ V}, E°_{Cu^{2+}/Cu} = +0.34 \text{ V}$$

With increasing voltage, the sequence of deposition of metals on the cathode will be:

A. Ag, Hg, Cu, Mg

B. Mg, Cu, Hg, Ag

C. Ag, Hg, Cu

D. Cu, Hg, Ag

Question 13

The following cell is set up:

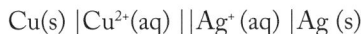

Cu(s) $|Cu^{2+}(aq)||Ag^+(aq)|Ag$ (s)

If the electrode potentials are

$Cu^{2+}/Cu=+0.34$ V and $Ag^+/Ag=+0.80$ V

What will be the e.m.f of the cell?

A. +1.14 V

B. +0.46 V

C. -0.46 V

D. -1.14 V

Question 14

Standard electrode potentials for the gain of one electron by the ions Cu^+ (aq) and Cu^{2+}(aq) are as follows:

$Cu^+(aq) +e^- \rightarrow Cu$ (s) $E° = + 0.52$ V

$Cu^{2+}(aq) +e^- \rightarrow Cu^+$ (s) $E° = + 0.16$ V

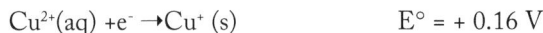

The standard reduction, in volts, for the disproportionate reaction,

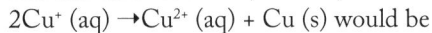

$2Cu^+$ (aq) $\rightarrow Cu^{2+}$ (aq) + Cu (s) would be

A. -0.68

B. -0.36

C. +0.36

D. +0.68

Question 15

A student set up the apparatus to determine the hydrogen ion concentration of solution X in the following cell

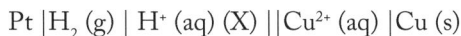

Pt $|H_2$ (g) $|$ H^+ (aq) (X) $||Cu^{2+}$ (aq) $|Cu$ (s)

The bridge was a glass tube filled with

A. Moist cotton wool

B. Cotton wool soaked in saturated KNO_3 solution

C. Cotton wool soaked in saturated copper sulfate solution

D. Cotton wool soaked in saturated sugar solution

Question 16

The values of the standard reduction potentials of the following reactions are given

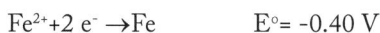

$Cu^{2+}+2e^- \rightarrow Cu$ $E°= +0.34$ V

$Sn^{2+}+2$ $e^- \rightarrow Sn$ $E°= -0.14$ V

$Zn^{2+}+2$ $e^- \rightarrow Zn$ $E°= -0.76$ V

$Fe^{2+}+2$ $e^- \rightarrow Fe$ $E°= -0.40$ V

Which one of the following is most easily reduced and oxidized?

A. Cu, Zn

B. Zn, Sn

C. Fe, Cu

D. Cu, Sn

Question 17

The standard reduction potential values of three metallic cations, X, Y, Z are 0.52, -3.03 and -1.18 V respectively. The order of reducing power of the corresponding metals is,

A. Y > Z >X

B. X > Y> Z

C. Z > Y> X

D. Z > X >Y

Solution

Question 1

STEP 1 = > What do you need to determine to solve the problem?
The amount of Al, Cu and Na deposited at the cathode in moles.

STEP 2 = > What relevant data provided in this problem is necessary in order to answer the question?
The amount of electricity passed is 1 Faraday. You also know M = ZIt, which says that the mass of an ion is equal to the electrochemical equivalent × the current × time. Also, it states Faraday's law which is that the weight deposited at an electrode = (I × t × gram equivalent weight of the substance deposited) / 96,500.

STEP 3 = > Use the relevant data to solve the question
In this case, you need to find the equivalent for each of the three metals, Al, Cu, and Na respectively.
One faraday will produce one equivalent each of:

For Al it is 3e⁻, for Cu it is 2e⁻, and for Na it is 1e⁻

Recall that the gram equivalent weight = m.wt./ the mole of electron gained or lost per mole of substance being oxidized or reduced.

$$= \frac{27}{3}; = \frac{64}{2}; = 23$$

=9g Al; 32g Cu; 23g Na are deposited.

Since 1 F = 96500 C and 1 C = 1 amp-s and these metals were deposited for 1 sec, the weight of the substance deposited at the electrode will be equal to the GEW of that substance.

Converting each to moles gives

1/3 mole Al, 1/2 mole Cu, and 1 mole Na

The answer is A.

Question 2

STEP 1 = > What do you need to determine to solve the problem?
The amount of Ni that can be deposited using the given parameters.

STEP 2 = > What relevant data provided in this problem is necessary in order to answer the question?
Given that certain current liberated 5.64 L hydrogen gas in 7.200×10^3 s
Also, atomic Mass of Ni = 59 gm

STEP 3 = > Use the relevant data to solve the question
First calculate the number of moles of H_2 in 5.64L using the gas equation at STP
(1 atm, 273K_

$$n = \frac{PV}{RT} = \frac{1atm(5.64L)}{(0.0821Latm/molK)(273K)}$$

n = 0.25 mol, the weight of H_2 is 0.50 g.
now, using Faraday's law, calculate the current you know
so that the $2H^+ \longrightarrow H_2 + 2e^-$

so $\quad M = \frac{Itz}{96500}$

$$0.50 = \frac{I(7.2 \times 10^3 s)(\frac{2}{2})}{96500}$$

I = 6.7A

$$Ni^{2+} + 2e^- \rightarrow Ni$$
$$2e^- \equiv 1 \text{ mol Ni} \equiv 59 \text{ g}$$

$$\therefore m = \frac{6.7(7.2 \times 10^3)(\frac{59}{2})}{96500}$$

m = 14.8g, answer A.

Question 3
STEP 1 = > What do you need to determine to solve the problem?
We have to find the amount of Ag and Zn that will be deposited.

STEP 2 = > What relevant data provided in this problem is necessary in order to answer the question?
The quantity of electricity passed is given = 0.200 mole e^-. You are also given the molecular weight of both silver and zinc.

STEP 3= > Use the relevant data to solve the question
The cathode reactions in the two electrolytic cells are

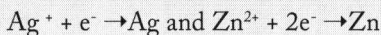

$$Ag^+ + e^- \rightarrow Ag \text{ and } Zn^{2+} + 2e^- \rightarrow Zn$$

The same amount of electricity (0.2F) has been passed through both the cells
Therefore,
Amount of silver deposited $= 108 \times 0.2 = 21.6g$

Amount of zinc deposited $\frac{65}{2} \times 0.2 = 6.5g$
The answer is C.

Question 4

STEP 1 = > What do you need to determine to solve the problem?
The amount of oxygen liberated under the given conditions.

STEP 2 = > What relevant data provided in this problem is necessary in order to answer the question?
It's given that 0.504 g of hydrogen is liberated in 2.00 hours.

STEP 3= > Use the relevant data to solve the question
Number of moles of H_2 liberated = 0.504/2= 0.252 mol.

The cathode reaction for the liberation of H_2 gas is

1 mol $H_2 \equiv$ 2 F

$\therefore$ 0.252 mol $H_2 \equiv$ 0.504 F

The reaction for the liberation of O_2 is

$2H_2O \rightarrow O_2 + 4H^+ + 4e^-$

$4F \equiv 1$ mol $O_2 \equiv 32g$

$\therefore$ 0.504 F will deposit 32×0.504/4 = 4.032g O_2

The answer is A.

Question 5

STEP 1 = > What do you need to determine to solve the problem?
The oxidation state of the tin in the salt has to be determined.

STEP 2 = > What relevant data provided in this problem is necessary in order to answer the question?
You are given that the current is 2.00 Amperes and the duration of current flow is 1.93×10^4 seconds. You are told that 23.8 g of tin is deposited.

STEP 3 = > Use the relevant data to solve the question
For finding the oxidation number, the number of moles of tin and the number of faradays are to be determined.

No. of faradays = 2.00 A × 1.93×10^4 s/ 96500 amp-s/F = 0.4 F (use conversions from chapter)

Number of moles of tin deposited = $\frac{23.8}{119} = 0.2$ mol Sn (using the given m.w. of Sn)

The oxidation state of Sn = $\frac{0.4}{0.2} = 2$

The answer is A.

Question 6

STEP 1 = > What do you need to determine to solve the problem?
We have to find the oxidizing agent in the reaction.

STEP 2 = > What relevant data is required for finding the oxidizing agent?
The equation of the reaction is given. You are also told that cations move towards the cathode and gain electrons. The battery pumps electrons into the cathode and reduction takes place.
$$A^+ + e^- \rightarrow A \text{ (reduction)}$$
The battery pumps electrons out of the anode, and substances capable of being oxidized (anions) give electrons up at the anode.

STEP 3 = > Use the relevant data to solve the question
Reduction is a decrease in the oxidation state and a gain of electrons. A substance that reduces itself acts as an oxidizing agent. In the reaction given, the oxidation state of Mn has charged from +7 in MnO_4^- to +2 in Mn^{2+}. Therefore, MnO_4^- has reduced itself to Mn^{2+} and acts as an oxidizing agent, answer is B.

Question 7

STEP 1 = > What do you need to determine to solve the problem?
We have to balance the charge.

STEP 2 = > What relevant data provided in this problem is necessary in order to answer the question?
The chemical reaction equation is given.

STEP 3 = > Use the relevant data to solve the question
Balance the charge on each species in the reaction
$$PbO_2 + 4H^+ + SO_4^{2-} + X \rightarrow PbSO_4 + 2H_2O$$

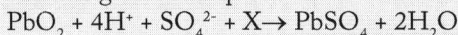

On the left side of the equation, in the first molecule, Pb has a charge of +4, O has a charge of −2, in the second the total is a charge of +4 for H, next you have an overall charge of −2 for the SO_4^{2-}.

On the right side, Pb has a charge of +2, SO_4^{2-} stays the same at −2, H stays the same at +4, and O stays the same at -2, so to balance the charge, we should add two electrons on the left, the answer is A.

Question 8

STEP 1 = > What do you need to determine to solve the problem?
You need to determine why stirring is essential.

STEP 2 = > What relevant data provided in this problem is necessary in order to answer the question?
You are told that you are reducing gold from the $AuCl_4^-$ ion and the solution must be stirred. Different options are given as to why this is necessary. You are also told that the

cations move towards the cathode and gain electrons. A battery pumps electrons into the cathode and reduction takes place.

STEP 3 = > Use the relevant data to solve the question
The answer is D. The $AuCl_4^-$ anion, which is negatively charged, must
be reduced at an electrode with excess electrons, also negatively charged. Since like charges repel, stirring is essential to get the anions to the electrode.

Question 9

STEP 1 = > What do you need to determine to solve the problem?
You need to determine which metal salt solution can be stored in the containers made of the other three metals.

STEP 2 = > What relevant data provided in this problem is necessary in order to answer the question?
The metals are given with their potentials for reduction.

STEP 3 = > Use the relevant data to solve the question
Al, Fe and Cu, are all weaker reducing agents than Mg indicated by the more negative value of the potential for reduction of Mg. As a result, none of these metals will reduce Mg^{2+} to Mg. Hence $MgSO_4$ solution can be stored safely in any one of these container. The answer is A.

Note that the question says the "metal container". Therefore we are looking for a "metal salt solution" that will not oxidize the other metal (cause the metal to lose electrons.
Thus looking at A. the metal salt solution would be $MgSO_4$
$Mg^{2+} + 2e^- \rightarrow Mg$

Then for this to be stable aluminium, iron and copper must not lose electrons if they come into contact with the Magnesium. Let's see some maths.

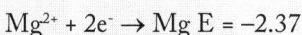

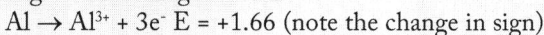

$Mg^{2+} + 2e^- \rightarrow Mg$ E = −2.37
$Al \rightarrow Al^{3+} + 3e^-$ E = +1.66 (note the change in sign)

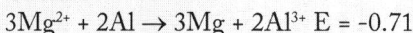

Overall:
$3Mg^{2+} + 2Al \rightarrow 3Mg + 2Al^{3+}$ E = -0.71
Not spontaneous because of the − E value. Since you get a -E value, there will be no oxidation. If you do the maths for the Fe and Cu, you will get −E values for both indicating that they are not spontaneous. If you reversed the reaction in all, you will get a spontaneous reaction; i.e. the metal salt solution will oxidize the metal container.

Question 10

STEP 1 = > What do you need to determine to solve the problem?
We have to find out the order of reactivity.

STEP 2 = > What relevant data provided in this problem is necessary in order to answer the question?
E° values of different cells are given.

STEP 3 = > Use the relevant data to solve the question
The reactivity of metal is defined as the tendency to lose electrons. The lower the electrode potential, the tendency to lose electrons increases as does the reactivity. The correct order of reactivity on the basis of E° value given is

Cu < Fe< Al < Mg
(Highest   (Lowest
E° value)   E° value)
The answer is B.

Question 11
STEP 1 = > What do you need to determine to solve the problem?
We have to find the strongest reducing agent.

STEP 2 = > What relevant data provided in this problem is necessary in order to answer the question?
E° values of different cells are given.

STEP 3 = > Use the relevant data to solve the question
The strongest reducing agent is one that has a lowest E° value. This makes Mg the strongest reducing agent. The answer is D.

Question 12
STEP 1 = > What do you need to determine to solve the problem?
The sequence of deposition of metals on the cathode.

STEP 2 = > What relevant data provided in this problem is necessary in order to answer the question?
The E° values of the different cells are given.

STEP 3 = > Use the relevant data to solve the question
The tendency for deposition at an electrode increases as E value increases
Therefore, the order will be Ag > Hg > Cu.
Silver has the highest reducing potential. Therefore it gains electrons the "easiest". The more positive the reduction potential the more likely it is for the first half reaction to occur. Although Mg^{2+} has a negative potential this is only the case relative to the hydrogen reduction potential as the numbers are an arbitrary way of evaluating this phenomena. Thus, if a voltage was applied (we are not trying to create a potential difference) to all (electron transfer and movement) then Mg^{2+} would be reduced too.

Because it has the highest reducing potential, Ag will deposit first and the Cu last. The answer is C. Mg will remain in the solution.

Question 13

STEP 1 = > What do you need to determine to solve the problem?
You need to find the $E°_{cell}$.

STEP 2 = > What relevant data provided in this problem is necessary in order to answer the question?
The individual E values are given.

STEP 3 = > Use the relevant data to solve the question
Remember, the cathode is always on the right, since the potentials are given both as reduction reactions. Therefore, the potential at the anode must be made negative because it is an oxidation reaction. Thus,

$$E°_{cell} = E°_{cathode} + E°_{anode}$$
$$= +0.80 + (-0.34)$$
$$= +0.46 \text{ V. The answer is B.}$$

Question 14

STEP 1 = > What do you need to determine to solve the problem?
You need to find the potential for the reduction of the disproportionate reaction

STEP 2 = > What relevant data provided in this problem is necessary in order to answer the question?
The individual E values are given

$Cu^+(aq) + e^- \rightarrow Cu (s)$	$E° = + 0.52$ V all superscripts and subscripts need to be in place
$Cu^{2+}(aq) + e^- \rightarrow Cu^+ (s)$	$E° = + 0.16$ V

STEP 3 = > Use the relevant data to solve the question

$Cu^+(aq) + e^- \rightarrow Cu (s)$	$E° = + 0.52$ V
$Cu^+(aq) \rightarrow Cu^{2+} (aq) + e^-$	$E° = - 0.16$ V
$2Cu^+ (aq) \rightarrow Cu^{2+} (aq) + Cu (s)$	$E° = ?$

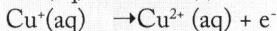
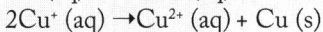

$$E°_{cell} = E°_{cathode} + E°_{anode}$$
$$= 0.52 - 0.16$$
$$= 0.36 \text{ V}$$

The answer is C.

Question 15

STEP 1 = > What do you need to determine to solve the problem?
You need to determine the salt bridge used.

STEP 2 = > What relevant data provided in this problem is necessary in order to answer the question?
The components of the cells are given.

Step 3 = > Use the relevant data to solve the question
The salt bridge must be composed of conducting ions that do not react with the solutions they connect. Aqueous potassium nitrate is a suitable chemical and the cotton wool will slow down mixing of the solution. The answer is B.

Question 16

STEP 1 = > What do you need to determine to solve the problem?
You have to find out the most easily reduced and most easily oxidized element.

STEP 2 = > What relevant data provided in this problem is necessary in order to answer the question?
The values of the standard reduction potentials of the metals are given.

STEP 3 = > Use the relevant data to solve the question
As the $E°$ value increases, the tendency to get reduced increases and the tendency to get oxidized decreases. Note that these are the reduction equations given. The larger the potential, the greater the tendency for the reaction to proceed. On the basis of $E°$ value given, we can say that Cu is the most easily reduced and Zn is the most easily oxidized. The answer is A.

Question 17

STEP 1 = > What do you need to determine to solve the problem?
The order of reducing power of the corresponding metals.

STEP 2 = > What relevant data provided in this problem is necessary in order to answer the question?
The standard reduction potential values of three metallic captions, X, Y, Z are 0.52, -3.03 and -1.18 V respectively.

STEP 3 = > Use the relevant data to solve the question
As $E°$ value decreases, the tendency to gain electrons by the metal ion decreases but the reducing power of the corresponding metal increases. The order of increasing reducing power is Y >Z > X which is given in answer A.

Chapter 9: **Chemical Kinetics**

> **Tip:** GAMSAT questions invariably include questions from chemical kinetics. If you can comprehend the basics of this topic, it's quite easy to score marks in the GAMSAT with questions in this topic.

Chemical kinetics is the study of the rates of reactions, the effect of reaction conditions on these rates and the mechanisms implied by such observations. At the macroscopic level we are interested in the amounts reacted, formed and the rates of their formation.

Key Concepts: Chemical Kinetics

Reaction Rate.

The rate of reaction is the change in concentration per unit time for a reactant or a product. It is the number of moles per litre of reactant particles disappearing, or the number of moles per litre of products being produced in a unit of time (molarity per second). Conventionally, the rate of disappearance of a reactant is taken as negative and the rate of appearance of a product as positive. Since the rate may vary with time, it is usual to define rate over a very small period of time Δt. It can be thought of as the derivative of concentration with respect to time or

$$rate = \frac{d[concentration]}{dt}$$

The derivative is the slope of a graph of concentration against time, taken at a particular time.

A number of factors can affect the **_rate of reaction._**

- o The nature of the reactants: acid-base reactions, salt formation, and ion exchange are fast reaction. Reactions that involve large molecules that are formed or break apart are usually slow. Reactions involving strong covalent bonds are also slow
- o Temperature: usually, the higher the temperature, the faster the reaction
- o Concentration Effect: the dependence of reaction rates on concentration are called rate law and will be discussed further in subsequent sections
- o Heterogeneous reactions: reactants are present in more than one phase, for these types of reactions, the rates are affected by surface area
- o Pressure: For solids and liquids the effect of pressure is negligible since they are essentially

incompressible. By increasing the pressure, gas molecules are forced to collide more often thereby increasing the rate of the reaction

o Surface area: If a reaction takes place at the boundary between two phases, the surface area will affect the rate. By increasing the surface area, effectively the number of molecules available to react is increased thereby increasing the rate of the reaction

o Catalysts: substances used to facilitate reactions

Rate Law

For almost all forward irreversible reactions, the rate is proportional to the product of the concentrations of the reactants, each raised to some power. For the general reaction

$$aA + bB \rightarrow cC$$

For the rate of reaction of the individual species, there will be a proportional relation between the disappearance of the reactants and the formation of the products, or more simply:

$$-\frac{1}{a}\frac{d[A]}{dt} = -\frac{1}{b}\frac{d[B]}{dt} = \frac{1}{c}\frac{d[C]}{dt}$$

The overall rate of the reaction will be proportional to $[A]^x[B]^y$, that is:

$$rate = k[A]^x[B]^y$$

The units for the rate of reaction will be obtained in *concentration/time.*

The exponents x and y are called the orders of the reaction and must be determined experimentally. These are not necessarily equal to the stoichiometric coefficients of the overall reaction.

The overall order of a reaction is defined as the sum of the exponents, in this case it is equal to x + y.

Order of Reaction.

Chemical reactions are often classified on the basis of first order, second order, mixed order or higher order reactions.

Consider the general reaction $aA + bB \rightarrow$ products.

1) Zero Order Reaction

A zero order reaction has a constant rate. It is independent of the reactant's concentration as shown:

$$rate = k$$

The rate constant for this type of reaction will have the units of mol L^{-1} s^{-1}

Photochemical reactions (in which the rate-determining factor is the light intensity, rather than the concentration of the reactant) are commonly zero order reactions.

2) First Order Reaction

A first order reaction has a rate of reaction proportional to the concentration of one of the reactants as shown:

$$\text{rate} = k\,[A]$$

The rate constant for this type of reaction will have units of $\sec^{-1}$.

As the reactant is consumed during this type of reaction, the concentration drops and so does the rate of reaction. The classic example of a first order reaction is radioactive decay where the concentration of the radioactive substance A can be expressed mathematically as shown:

$$[A_t] = [A_o]e^{-kt}$$

where:

$[A_o]$ = initial concentration of A

$[A_t]$ = concentration of A at time t

k = rate constant

t = elapse time

A few examples of first order reactions with their rate equations are listed below:

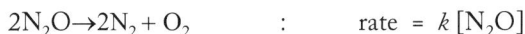

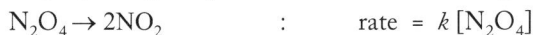

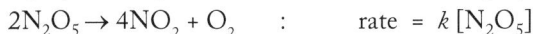

$$2N_2O \rightarrow 2N_2 + O_2 \qquad : \qquad \text{rate} = k\,[N_2O]$$

$$SO_2Cl_2 \rightarrow SO_2 + Cl_2 \qquad : \qquad \text{rate} = k\,[SO_2Cl_2]$$

$$N_2O_4 \rightarrow 2NO_2 \qquad : \qquad \text{rate} = k\,[N_2O_4]$$

$$2N_2O_5 \rightarrow 4NO_2 + O_2 \qquad : \qquad \text{rate} = k\,[N_2O_5]$$

3) Second-Order Reaction

A second order reaction has a rate proportional to the product of the concentration of two reactants or to the square of the concentration of a single reactant as shown:

$$\text{Rate} = k[A][B] = k[A]^2 = k[B]^2$$

The rate constant for this type of reaction will have units of L mol^{-1} s^{-1}.

In this type of reaction, as the concentration of the reactant increases, the rate of reaction increases rapidly. For example, when the concentration of the reactant is doubled, the rate will be quadrupled.

Practice Questions

Question 1-5

Consider the following reaction:

A + B$\rightarrow$ Products,

The rate equation for this reaction is r = k [A]^m [B]^n

Where m is the order of the reaction with respect to reagent A and n is the order of the reaction with respect to reagent B. Thus, the overall order of this reaction is m + n.

1. In an experiment to study the reaction A+2B $\rightarrow$C+2D, the initial rate of reagent A, r_A at t= 0 was found to be 2.6 $\times$ 10^{-2} Ms^{-1}. What is the rate of reagent B r_B at t=0 in Ms^{-1}?

    A. 2.6 $\times$ 10^{-2}

    B. 5.2 $\times$ 10^{-2}

    C. 1.3 $\times$ 10^{-2}

    D. 1.0 $\times$ 10^{-1}

2. In the reaction N_2 (g) + 3H_2 (g) $\rightarrow$2NH_3, the rate of formation of NH_3 will be

    A. the same as the rate of disappearance of N_2

    B. twice the rate of disappearance of N_2

    C. half the rate of disappearance of H_2

    D. the same as the rate of disappearance of H_2

3. If concentrations are measured in moles per litre and time in minutes, the data given units for the specific rate constant of a third-order reaction is

    A. mol L^{-1} min^{-1}

    B. L^2 mol^{-2} min^{-1}

    C. mol^2 L^{-2} min^{-1}

    D. min^{-1}

4. For the reaction X+Y →Z, the rate of reaction is expressed by
Rate = k[X]² [Y]^{1/2} , If the concentrations of X and Y are both increased by a factor of 4, by what factor will the rate increase?

  A. 4

  B. 8

  C. 16

  D. 32

5. The rate of reaction between X and Y is a third order overall. Which of the following rate equation must be INCORRECT?

  A. rate = k [X] [Y]³

  B. rate = k [X]² [Y] [Z]⁰

  C. rate = k [X]² [Y]

  D. rate = k [X]⁰ [Y]³

Solution

NOTE: In order to easily answer these questions, follow the three-step method described below.

Question 1

STEP 1 = > What do you need to determine to solve the problem?
For this problem we need to determine the value of r_B at t=0.

STEP 2 = > What relevant data provided in this problem is necessary in order to answer the question?
The initial rate of A, r_A at t= 0 is given.

STEP 3 = > Use this relevant data to solve the question
The equation which relate the disappearance of A and rate of disappearance of B is

$$-\frac{d[A]}{dt} = -\frac{1}{2} \times \frac{d[B]}{dt}$$

The rate of disappearance of B

$$= -\frac{d[B]}{dt} = 2\left|\frac{d[A]}{dt}\right|$$

$$= 2 \times 2.6 \times 10^{-2} = 5.2 \times 10^{-2} \, Ms^{-1}$$

The answer is B.

Question 2

STEP 1 = > What do you need to determine to solve the problem?
You are looking for the correct ratio of the rate of formation of NH_3 in relation to the reactants.

STEP 2 = > What relevant data provided in this problem is necessary in order to answer the question?
The chemical equation provided will be needed. It tells you how the relationship between different chemical species are consumed and produced.

STEP 3 = > Use the relevant data to solve the question
From the following equation N_2 (g) + $3H_2$ (g) $\rightarrow 2NH_3$, we know that during this reaction there will be 3 H_2 molecules consumed for every 1 N_2 molecule, thus the rate of disappearance of these two molecules will relate as follows:

$$-\frac{d[N_2]}{dt} = -\frac{1}{3} \times \frac{d[H_2]}{dt}$$

In addition, when 1 N_2 and 3 H_2 molecules are consumed, 2 NH_3 molecules will be formed thus giving the rate equations

$$-\frac{d[N_2]}{dt} = -\frac{1}{3} \times \frac{d[H_2]}{dt} = \frac{1}{2} \times \frac{d[NH_3]}{dt}$$

by multiplying each side of the equation by 2, the relationship between the disappearance of the two reagents and the formation of NH_3 can be determined.

Thus, the rate of NH_3 formation will be 2/3 times the rate of disappearance of H_2 as shown;

$$-\frac{2}{3} \times \frac{d[H_2]}{dt} = \frac{d[NH_3]}{dt}$$

And the rate of NH_3 formation will be 2 times the rate of N_2 disappearance as shown;

$$-2\frac{d[N_2]}{dt} = \frac{d[NH_3]}{dt}$$

This makes statement B the correct answer.

Question 3

STEP 1 = > What do you need to determine to solve the problem?
The units of k.

STEP 2 = > What relevant data provided in this problem is necessary in order to answer the question?
The order of the reaction is given.

STEP 3 = > Use the relevant data to solve the question
The units of any n^{th} order reaction can be determined by using the equation
$(mol)^{1-n}$ (vol. in L)$^{n-1}$ time^{-1}

For a third order reaction, n= 3.
$(mol)^{1-3}$ (L)$^{3-1}$ min^{-1} = mol^{-2} L^2 min^{-1}
Therefore, the answer is B.

Question 4

STEP 1 = > What do you need to determine to solve the problem?
You need to figure out by what factor the rate of reaction increases by.

STEP 2 = > What relevant data provided in this problem is necessary in order to answer the question?
The equation for the rate of the reaction is given. Therefore, you know the order of the equation since it is equal to the sum of the exponents.

STEP 3 = > Use the relevant data to solve the question
The order of the reaction can be calculated by adding the exponents – in this case the order is 2.5. The factor by which the reaction will increase in relation to the increasing concentration can be calculated by raising the factor by which the concentration increased to the power of the order. In this case, the factor of increase in concentration is 4 and the reaction has an order of 2.5, thus, $4^{2.5}$ = 32. Therefore, the answer is D.

Question 5

STEP 1 = > What do you need to determine to solve the problem?
You need to choose the incorrect option among the choices.

STEP 2 = > What relevant data provided in this problem is necessary in order to answer the question?
The order of the reaction is given.

STEP 3 = > Use the relevant data to solve the question
Remember, the order of the reaction is determined by adding the exponents of the concentrations. So, lets examine the choices, answer B) 2 + 1 + 0 = 3 – this is a 3rd order reaction; answer C) 2 + 1 = 3 – this is a 3rd order reaction; answer D) 0 + 3 = 3 – again, this is a 3rd order reaction; answer A) 1 + 3 = 4 - The answer is A, because the sum of the exponents is 4 making it a 4th order reaction. The correct answer is A.

GAMSAT Style Questions

Question 1

For a first order reaction $[A] = [A]_0 e^{-kt}$, the rate decreases exponentially with time. Which graph represents the plot of rate of reaction against time for a first order reaction?

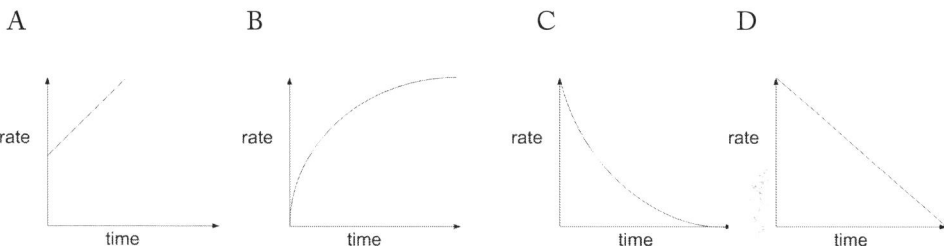

A   B   C   D

Question 2

When copper carbonate is reacted with excess acid, carbon dioxide is produced. The curves shown were obtained under different conditions.

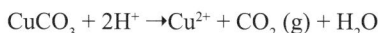

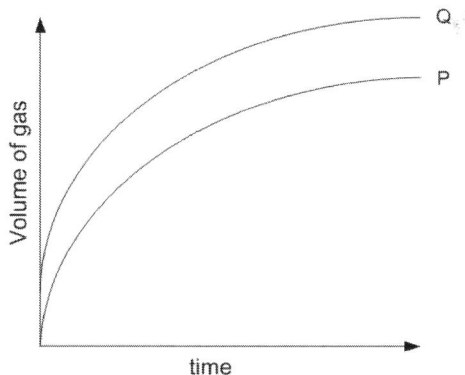

$$CuCO_3 + 2H^+ \rightarrow Cu^{2+} + CO_2\,(g) + H_2O$$

The change from P to Q could be brought about by

    A. increasing the concentration of the acid

    B. decreasing the mass of copper carbonate

    C. carrying out the reaction at a higher temperature

    D. adding a catalyst

Question 3

The rate equation for the reaction

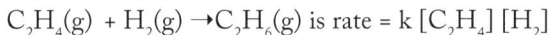

$$C_2H_4(g) + H_2(g) \rightarrow C_2H_6(g) \text{ is rate} = k\,[C_2H_4]\,[H_2]$$

If, at a fixed temperature, the reaction mixture is compressed to three times the original pressure, which one of the following is the factor by which the rate of reaction changes?

A. 3

B. 6

C. 9

D. 12

Question 4

For the reaction between chlorine and nitric oxide,

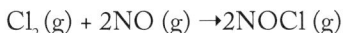

$$Cl_2(g) + 2NO(g) \rightarrow 2NOCl(g)$$
$$r = k[Cl_2]^x\,[NO]^y$$

It is found that doubling the concentration of both reactants increases the rate by a factor of 8. If only the concentration of Cl_2 is doubled, the rate increases by a factor of 2. What is the order of this reaction with respect to NO?

A. 0

B. 1

C. 2

D. 3

Question 5

The reaction A (g) +2B (g) →C (g) + D (g) is an elementary process where the rate is first order with respect to A and second order with respect to B. In an experiment, the initial partial pressures of A and B are P_A = 0.60 atm, and P_B = 0.80 atm, When P_C = 0.20 atm (P_A = 0.40 atm; P_B = 0.40 atm), the rate of the reaction, relative to the initial rate, is

A. $\dfrac{1}{24}$

B. $\dfrac{1}{16}$

C. $\dfrac{3}{4}$

D. $\dfrac{1}{6}$

Question 6

Two colourless substances X and Y react to give a coloured substance Z. The time (t) taken for various initial concentrations of X and Y to produce a certain colour in Z intensity are recorded in the table.

[X]/mol L^{-1}	[Y]/mol L^{-1}	Time /sec
0.05	0.05	44
0.05	0.10	22
0.10	0.05	44

Which rate equation is consistent with these results?

A. rate = k[Y]$^{1/2}$

B. rate = k [X]$^{1/2}$ [Y]$^{1/2}$

C. rate = k [Y]

D. rate = k [X] [Y]

Question 7 - 10

The rate equation for the rate of reaction can be given by,

$$r = k [A]^x [B]^y$$

For the reaction between acetone and iodine in the presence of hydrochloric acid (shown below)

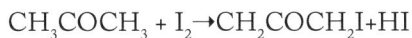

$$CH_3COCH_3 + I_2 \rightarrow CH_2COCH_2I + HI$$

the rate expression is given by

$$rate = k [CH_3COCH_3][H^+]$$

7. What is the overall order of the reaction?

A. Zero

B. One

C. Two

D. Three

8. A solution of Q_2 of concentration 0.20 mol L^{-1} undergoes a first order reaction at an initial rate of 3.0×10^{-4} mol L^{-1} s^{-1}. Calculate the rate constant.

     A. 6.0×10^{-3} s^{-1}

     B. 1.5×10^{-4} s^{-1}

     C. 0.60×10^{-3} s^{-1}

     D. 1.5×10^{-3} s^{-1}

9. For the reaction A+B →C, the following results were obtained for kinetic 'runs' at the same temperature:

$[A]_0$/mol L^{-1}	$[B]_0$/mol L^{-1}	Initial rate / mol L-1 s-1
0.20	0.10	0.20
0.40	0.10	0.80
0.40	0.20	0.80

What is the overall order of the reaction?

     A. 0

     B. 1

     C. 2

     D. 3

10. Which of the following statements is true?

     A. The rate constant of a first order reaction has units of mol L^{-1} sec^{-1}

     B. For a zero order reaction, the rate is independent of the concentration of the reactant

     C. For a zero order reaction, $t_{1/2} = \dfrac{0.693}{k}$

     D. The radio disintegration of uranium is a zero order reaction.

Question 11 – 13

The thermal decomposition of dinitrogen pentoxide, N_2O_5: can be expressed as $2N_2O_5(g) \rightarrow 4\ NO_2(g) + O_2(g)$. Assume the rate is the change per unit time. Given that, A is the average rate at which N_2O_5 disappears over the time interval from 1200s to 9600s. B is the average rate at which N_2O_5 disappears over the time interval from 3600 to 7200s. Consider average rate as the ratio of the change in concentration to the duration in seconds.

The data obtained during such a reaction is given below.

Decomposition of N_2O_5 at 45°C		
Time/s	$[N_2O_5]$/mol L^{-1}	$[O_2]$ /mol L^{-1}
600	0.0124	0.00254
1200	0.00932	0.00410
2400	0.00529	0.00612
3600	0.00292	0.00730
5400	0.00121	0.00816
7200	0.00050	0.00851
9600	0.00015	0.00871

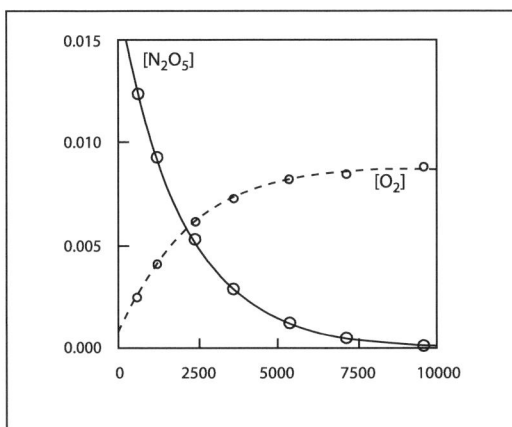

11. Considering the process between 1200 and 7200s, which of the following statements can be inferred? When the concentration of O_2 increases by 0.00441 mol L^{-1}

   A. The change in N_2O_5 concentration is twice as large as the change in O_2 concentration.

   B. The change in N_2O_5 concentration is equal to the change in O_2 concentration

   C. The change in N_2O_5 concentration is half of that of the change in O_2 concentration.

   D. The change in N_2O_5 concentration is four times as large as the change in O_2 concentration.

12. Considering the average rate, what is the relationship between the change in concentration of N_2O_5 from 1200 to 9600s and the change from 3600 to 7200s?

    A. 1.09:1

    B. 0.067:1

    C. 1:1.6

    D. 1:0.6

13. From the given data we can infer that between 600s and 1200s,

    A. The average rate of reaction for a specific period of N_2O_5 is double that of O_2

    B. The average rate of reaction for a specific period of O_2 is double that of N_2O_5

    C. The average rate of reaction for a specific period of O_2 is the same as that of N_2O_5

    D. The average rate of reaction for a specific period of O_2 is one-fourth that of N_2O_5

Question 14

14. For the reaction $2A + B \rightarrow C + D$, $-\frac{d[A]}{dt} = k[A]^2[B]$. The expression for the disappearance of B will be

    A. $k[A]^2[B]$

    B. $2k[A]^2[B]$

    C. $k[2A]^2[B]$

    D. $\frac{1}{2}k[A]^2[B]$

Solution

Question 1

STEP 1 = > What do you need to determine to solve the problem?
You have to select the right graph from the given possibilities.

STEP 2 = > What relevant data provided in this problem is necessary in order to answer the question?
Examining the given equation shows that the rate decreases exponentially.

STEP 3 = > Use the relevant data to solve the question
For a first order reaction, the rate of the reaction will be directly proportional to the concentration, and the concentration decreases exponentially with time. The graphic representation of an exponential decrease in concentration will be represented with an initial rapid decrease in the rate, which begins to level off as the time increases and the rate approaches zero. This is correctly represented in graph C.

Question 2

STEP 1 = > What do you need to determine to solve the problem?
We have to find out the method by which we can attain the plot Q from plot P, given in the graph.

STEP 2 = > What relevant data provided in this problem is necessary in order to answer the question?
The corresponding chemical reaction equation is given. In addition, a graphical representation of gas volume over time for the given reaction is provided. The graph shows the progression of the chemical reaction resulting in the production of carbon dioxide under two different undefined conditions. This graph demonstrates that as the reaction progresses over time, the amount of CO_2 first increases rapidly, and then production begins to slow. P demonstrates a proportionally overall lower amount of gas produced at all times than Q.

STEP 3 = > Use the relevant data to solve the question

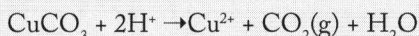

$$CuCO_3 + 2H^+ \rightarrow Cu^{2+} + CO_2(g) + H_2O$$

To understand this question, you need to understand what effects different components can have on the progression of a chemical reaction. The graph of P demonstrates a proportionally overall lower amount of gas produced at all times than Q. A catalyst would not produce more gas, but the same amount faster. Increasing temperature has a similar effect, since increasing temperature results in an increase in the kinetic energy of the molecules and thus more collisions causing the rate of the reaction to increase. It will not have any effect on the amount of gas produced. A decrease in the amount of $CuCO_3$ logically would have the opposite effect, since with less reactant, less product can be formed, so the volume of gas produced would be less. Therefore, an increase in the volume of gas produced in a given time can be accomplished by increasing the concentration of the acid, making A the correct answer.

HELPFUL HINT: Go through the process of elimination such as to why the other answers are wrong. This gives people the edge over others who do not know principles and basic knowledge.

Question 3

STEP 1 = > What do you need to determine to solve the problem?
The change in the rate of the equation under the given conditions has to be determined.

STEP 2 = > What relevant data provided in this problem is necessary in order to answer the question?
The chemical equation and the corresponding rate equation are given.

STEP 3 = > Use the relevant data to solve the question

$$Rate\ (r) = k\ [C_2H_4]\ [H_2]$$

When the reaction mixture compressed to three times, then new concentration of the reactants represented by the ' notation' will be

$$[C_2H_4]' = \frac{1}{3}[C_2H_4]$$

$$[H_2]' = \frac{1}{3}[H_2]$$

The new rate $r' = k\ [C_2H_4]'\ [H_2]' = \frac{1}{9}[C_2H_4][H_2]$

$$9r' = r$$

The rate will change by a factor of 9. The answer is C.

Question 4

STEP 1 = > What do you need to determine to solve the problem?
We have to find the order of the given reaction with respect to NO.

STEP 2 = > What relevant data provided in this problem is necessary in order to answer the question?
The effect of increasing the concentration of both reactants on the overall rate of reaction AND the effect of increasing the Cl_2 concentration on the overall reaction rate is given.

STEP 3 = > Use the relevant data to solve the question
Let the rate equation be $r = k\ [Cl_2]^x\ [NO]^y$
Where

$\qquad$ x = Order w.r.t Cl_2

$\qquad$ y = Order w.r.t NO

$\qquad$ $8r = k\ [2Cl_2]^x\ [2NO]^y$

$8r = 2^{x+y} r$

Or $2^{x+y} = 2^3$

Or $x+y = 3$

When only the concentration of Cl_2 is doubled, the rate increases by a factor of 2.

$2r = k (2Cl_2) x (NO)y$

$2r = 2xr$

$2x = 2$

$\therefore \quad x = 1$

Substituting x=1 equation (1) gives y=2

The order of this reaction with respect to (NO) = 2

The answer is C.

Question 5

STEP 1 = > What do you need to determine to solve the problem?

We have to find out the rate of the reaction, relative to the initial rate.

STEP 2 = > What relevant data provided in this problem is necessary in order to answer the question?

The reaction equation as well as the partial pressures is given.

STEP 3 = > Use the relevant data to solve the question

For an elementary process A (g) + 2B (g) →C (g) + D (g)

	A (g) +	2B (g) +	→C (g) +	D (g)
T = 0	0.60 atm	0.80 atm	0 atm	0 atm

(1) $r = k (0.60) (0.80)^2$

at t=t_1 0.40 atm   0.40 atm   0.20 atm

(2) $r' = k (0.40) (0.40)^2$

Dividing eq (2) by eq (1) give

$\dfrac{r'}{r} = \dfrac{1}{6}$ or $r' = \dfrac{1}{6}r$

The answer is D.

Question 6

STEP 1 = > What do you need to determine to solve the problem?
The rate equation that matches with the given data set needs to be determined.

STEP 2 = > What relevant data provided in this problem is necessary in order to answer the question?
The concentrations given at each time represent the amount each reactant (X and Y). In the first row, similar initial concentrations of X and Y are used and the resulting time to get a certain concentration of Z produced is recorded. In the second row, the concentration of X is held constant, while the concentration of Y is doubled and again the time is recorded to get that same concentration of Z. In the last row of data, the concentration of X is doubled while the concentration of Y is held constant.

STEP 3 = > Use the relevant data to solve the question
When the concentration of Y is doubled between the first and second reading, the time halves, and hence rate doubles. Therefore, the reaction must be first order with respect to Y. However, when the concentration of X is doubled, there is no effect on the time and hence the rate of reaction remains the same. The reaction must be zero order with respect to X since concentration has no effect on the rate of reaction. The equation that shows a rate that is first order with respect to Y and zero order with respect to X is shown in answer C.

Question 7

STEP 1 = > What do you need to determine to solve the problem?
We have to find out the overall order of the reaction.

STEP 2 = > What relevant data provided in this problem is necessary in order to answer the question?
The rate equation for the reaction is given demonstrating that the rate is dependant on the concentrations of the reactants each raised to the first power.

STEP 3 = > Use the relevant data to solve the question
$$r = k\,[CH_3COCH_3]\,[H^+]$$
The exponent of acetone =1 and that of H^+ is also 1. Since the overall order of the reaction is equal to the sum of the exponents, the rate is equal to $1 + 1 = 2$. The answer is C.

Question 8

STEP 1 = > What do you need to determine to solve the problem?
The rate constant is to be determined

STEP 2 = > What relevant data provided in this problem is necessary in order to answer the question?
The order of the reaction is given as a first order reaction and the initial rate (r) is provided. The value of the concentration of solution [Q] is provided as well.

STEP 3 = > Use the relevant data to solve the question

Since this is a first order reaction, the rate equation is

$R = k[Q]$

$$k = \frac{r}{[Q]} = \frac{3.0 \times 10^{-4}\, molL^{-1}s^{-1}}{0.20molL^{-1}} R = k[Q]$$

$$= 1.5 \times 10^{-3}\, s^{-1}$$

The answer is D.

Question 9

STEP 1 = > What do you need to determine to solve the problem?

We have to determine the rate of the equation.

STEP 2 = > What relevant data provided in this problem is necessary in order to answer the question?

The effect on rate of doubling each reactant is provided. In the second row of data, the effect on reaction rate of doubling the concentration of A is demonstrated, and in the third row, the effect of doubling the concentration of B is shown.

STEP 3 = > Use the relevant data to solve the question

Let the rate eqn. be r = k [A] ^{x} [B]^y

Where x = order w.r.t [A] and y = order w.r.t [B]

We have   0.20 = k (0.20) ^{x} (0.10) ^{y}

0.80 = k (0.40) ^{x} (0.10) ^{y}

0.80 = k (0.40) ^{x} (0.20) ^{y}

Dividing eqn (2) by (1) give   x = 2

Dividing eqn (3) by (2) give   y = 0

The answer is C.

Question 10

STEP 1 = > What do you need to determine to solve the problem?

The correct statement among the choices has to be determined.

STEP 2 = > What relevant data provided in this problem is necessary in order to answer the question?

The rate equation is given, it shows that any reaction rate with exponents of zero would be independent of concentration.

STEP 3 = > Use the relevant data to solve the question

The only true statement is B – if the order is zero, the exponents would be zero and therefore the rate would be independent of concentration.

The first statement is wrong because k has units of s^{-1}

$$t_{1/2} = \frac{0.693}{k}$$

is half-life for a first order reaction not a zero order reaction
The radio disintegration reaction follows first order kinetics.

Question 11

STEP 1 = > What do you need to determine to solve the problem?
The change in the concentration of N_2O_5 and O_2 has to be determined.

STEP 2 = > What relevant data provided in this problem is necessary in order to answer the question?
We have been provided with both a graph and the table. Since you can retrieve the necessary given data from the table rather than the graph, concentrate on the table.

STEP 3 = > Use the relevant data to solve the question
When the concentration of N_2O_5 decreases by 0.00882 mol L^{-1} (*i.e.* (0.00932 – 0.00050) mol L^{-1}) between 1200 and 7200s, the concentration of O_2 increases by 0.00441 mol L^{-1}. Hence the answer is A.

Question 12

STEP 1 = > What do you need to determine to solve the problem?
The ratio of the average rate between two given intervals has to be determined.

STEP 2 = > What relevant data provided in this problem is necessary in order to answer the question??
The concentration of N_2O_5 at different time points is provided.

STEP 3 = > Use the relevant data to solve the question

Average rate = $\dfrac{[N_2O_5]_{t=9600s} - [N_2O_5]_{t=1200s}}{9600s - 1200s}$

Average rate = $\dfrac{(0.00015 - 0.00932)molL^{-1}}{(9600 - 1200)s}$

Average rate = -1.09×10^{-6} mol L^{-1} s^{-1}

For the second interval,

Average rate = $\dfrac{[N_2O_5]_{t=7200s} - [N_2O_5]_{t=3600s}}{7200s - 3600s}$

Average rate = -0.672×10^{-6} mol L^{-1} s^{-1}

Hence the ratio is 1.09:0.67 = 1:0.6, answer D.

Question 13

Consider the period 600-1200s
Use the same steps as described in Question 12

Average Rate for O_2 = 0.00254 – 0.00410 = – 0.00156 mol $L^{-1}s^{-1}$
Average Rate for N_2O_5 = 0.0124 – 0.00932 = + 0.00308 mol $L^{-1}s^{-1}$
Hence the answer is A.

Question 14

STEP 1 = > What do you need to determine to solve the problem?
An expression for the disappearance of B.

STEP 2 = > What relevant data provided in this problem is necessary in order to answer the question?
The general reaction equation is given, as is the rate equation.

STEP 3 = > Use the relevant data to solve the question
For the reaction 2A+B→ C+D, we have

$$-\frac{1}{2} \times \frac{d[A]}{dt} = -\frac{d[B]}{dt}$$

$$\therefore \quad \frac{d[B]}{dt} = \frac{1}{2} \times \frac{d[A]}{dt} = \frac{1}{2}k[A]2[B]$$

The answer is D.

Printed in Great Britain
by Amazon